Best Nutritional Health With An Alkaline Body

"Use Vegetables and Fruits To Eliminate Illness"

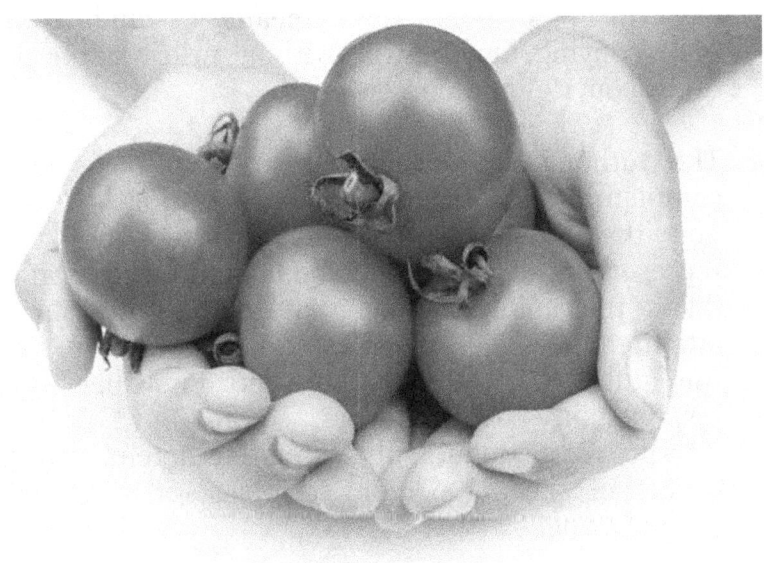

Rudy S Silva, Natural Nutritionist

TABLE OF CONTENTS

Chapter 1: Introduction

Super Health

One of the ways to maintain better health is to eat more clean or organic fruits and vegetables and less protein, fat and carbohydrates. There is just no way around this. The purpose of eating more produce is to provide the nutrients your body needs to keep disease away, to detoxify your body, and to maintain your body in an alkaline condition.

To maintain health and keep disease away you must eat the food that provides you with the most nutrition and which does the least damage to your body. You want to eat the foods that have high nutrition and which are the lowest in protein, carbohydrates, fat, sugar, and calories.

What is happening to people with disease is they are eating more than they need of everything they find in a grocery store. If you are overweight and want to lose weight, you have to do the opposite of what got you obese – eat less protein, carbohydrates, fat, sugar, and calories. All terminal diseases are cause by what we eat and how much we eat of that food.

Eating the wrong foods and too much of them results in a nutritional deficiency and disease.

If you change your eating habits to mainly include nutritious foods, expect to gain these benefits: live a long life, slow down your aging, create a strong immune system, prevent disease, and have super health to enjoy your life.

Toxic Body

Most people have a toxic body. This comes from all the contamination that is in the air, food, popular drinks, and water. Contamination or pollution has a destructive action in your body. It is filled with free radicals that combine with your body's tissue forming an inflammation, which later turns into a specific disease – arthritis, arteriosclerosis, erectile dysfunction, Alzheimer's, senility, skin cancers, and so on.

There is really no way to stop pollution, all you can do is protect yourself with antioxidants that help you neutralize it. You can also on occasion do a body cleanse to suck out toxins that result from pollution and to clean out the colon where most diseases come from. A body cleanse can pull out toxic matter and pathogens out of your body.

Acid Body

It is well known now that when your body fluids are acidic, you will be prone to more illness and disease. First of all, acid in your body creates inflammation. It's this inflammation, that you don't feel, which slowly leads to the deterioration of your organs and tissue. This is why as you age, you can start to see the appearance of various diseases in your body. In some cases, you will see the results of your acid body in the conditions it creates - gout, arthritis, muscle fatigue, acid reflux, bone loss, heart conditions, respiratory conditions, and many more conditions.

Various pathogens like an acid environment and setup

household in your body. As these pathogens, bacteria, viruses, and parasite multiple, they make your body more acidic, because of their excretions. As your body weakens, these pathogens become more established in your body. As you weaken further, the pathogens destroy cells, and tissue on various surfaces or organs in your body, leading to multiple diseases.

Fruits and Vegetables

The secret to having good health is to have a diet that is properly balance with fruits, vegetables, carbohydrates and protein and fat. But, to get to the point where a balanced diet can have the wanted health benefits, you need to do some changes in the way you eat and live.

Because your body is probably out of balance, you need to get it back into balance. And, you cannot do it simply by eating a good diet. If you have illnesses, you need to get rid of them, using natural remedies. Then you need to follow a healthy lifestyle, so that you can rebalance your body. It takes about a year or more to rebalance your body.

In the following chapters, you will find a direction and information that you can use to rebalance your body and improve your health. You cannot simple start eating fruits and vegetables in normal quantities and expect to become healthy. You have to over eat or over supplement with those things that will help. This will give your body an excess of the nutrients it needs to overcome any deteriorated condition your body has.

One of the first things you want to do is to make your body more alkaline. This means removing the excess acid your body has. Here is how you can start to make your body more alkaline.

1. Do a short body and blood cleanse

2. Get in tune with your body cycles. The body cycles help you normalize your hormones, revitalize your cells and tissue, and remove toxic waste from your body.

3. Eat more fruits and vegetables.

4. Measure your body pH to track your acid and alkaline body conditions.

5. Take certain supplements that help your body recover from illness and body damage.

This e-book does not cover the exercise you need to do, but you do need to do some exercise to have the best health. So find a program that you feel comfortable with and do it regularly. One of the best exercise programs I have found is called PACE. You can search on the internet for this program.

CHAPTER 2: ACID ALKALINE pH BODY TEST

Acid Binding Minerals

Moving your body more toward alkalinity is what will give you the best curative effects of fruits and vegetables. An alkaline body prevents your body from becoming ill and forming deadly diseases, like all kinds of joint problems, organ degradation, body pain, heart disease or even cancer. If you are already sick, then all of the chemicals inside fruits will help to revive you to better health. This is provided that your tissue damage has not gone beyond repair.

The minerals most important in changing and maintaining your body in an alkaline condition are sodium, potassium, chloride, calcium, phosphorus, magnesium, and sulfur.

Now, how your body can become alkaline might become a little confusing at first because of the terms used, but let's break this down into small parts. First we are going to be defining some terms so we can then start talking the same language.

Acid Binding

There are certain minerals that are called acid binding. And these are minerals we said are the most important ones in fruits and vegetables, Sodium, potassium, chloride, calcium, phosphorus, magnesium, because they are acid binding.

What acid binding means is when you eat produce with these minerals, your cells create what is called **Alkaline Forming Ash**. This ash seeks out acids in your body and combines with them to neutralize them.

Alkaline Forming Ash

Now, this alkaline forming ash has the ability to tie up an acid and carried to the kidney, where it is expelled as urine. There are other exit points for this neutralized acid and this is provided by the other three channels of elimination – lungs, colon, and skin.

Acids in your body are toxic, so the body has the priority of getting rid of them fast, since they can damage tissue and cause pain and disease. It can do this fast as long as you have plenty of alkaline forming ash in your body.

Different reactions can occur when alkaline ash mineral, like say sodium, encounters an acid. Here is another path way of the acid neutralization process when it combines with alkaline ash.

The Acid Binding Mineral Process

When you eat acid binding food, fruits and vegetables, the blood carries them into your cells where it is oxidized, digested, or metabolized. The result of this digestion is a carbonic acid salt of alkaline minerals, which reacts with body acids and binds with them.

In this process, a weak carbonic acid is created. Now, this weak carbonic acid is taken by the blood into the lungs where it is released as carbon dioxide and water.

If not all the acid toxins are captured by alkaline ash, the remaining acids can be neutralized by the body's stores of alkaline minerals. If you don't have a good store of alkaline minerals within your body, then these acids will remain in your body creating damage and disease. But if you do have a good store of alkaline minerals, then these minerals will find these acids, capture them and bind with them. These acids are then eliminated through your urine and out of your body.

Body Acids

You may be wondering where do these body acids come from? Body acids are created from many sources. When you eat meat and it is digested and metabolized by your cells, the residue will be an acid. When you smoke or breathe polluted air, your body will accumulate acids. When you eat junk food, the additives, such as dyes, preservatives, and enhancers, will create acid. When you are stress or have strong negative thoughts, this will create body acids. When you exercise, you will create acids. There are so many foods or conditions that can create acids in your body.

Alkaline reserves

If you have depleted the alkaline ash that is available and still have acid in your body, this causes your body to dip into your alkaline store reserves to neutralize this acid. If your reserves are depleted then, your body will borrow minerals - sodium, magnesium, calcium, and potassium - from bones and vital organs to effectively neutralize the acid and remove it from your body safely. This is what causes disease.

The alkaline reserve is a back-up system, with limited quantity to keep you from constantly poisoning yourself with too much acid-forming food, bad habits, and exercise. When there is overindulgence in acid-forming foods, especially fried and junk food your body becomes sick.

In its marvelous wisdom, the body will make every possible effort to rebalance your acid body by removing acids as quickly as possible. But, when you constantly deplete your alkaline reserves and you don't eat enough alkaline forming food – fruits and vegetables, you will develop terminal diseases.

Achieving alkaline balance in your body consists of eating 80% alkaline forming foods and 20% acid forming.

So you can see the importance of getting a lot of alkaline minerals into your body. Without them, acids, which do not get bonded to an alkaline minerals would move back into body tissue and continue their body damage.

Measure Body Acidity

Measuring your overall body acidity is difficult to do, since there are no diagnostic tests that can easily do this. There are some pH tests that you can do that will give you a relative indication of what your body's pH is at a specific moment. For this test you need pH litmus paper.

pH Explained

pH – is a complex mathematical and chemical system that was developed to determine when a liquid or solution is an acid or base. Its definition is:

"The negative logarithm of the hydrogen ion molarity"

Since the pH scale is logarithmic, each whole pH value along its scale is ten times stronger. So pH 6.0 is ten time more acidic than pH 7.0 and pH 5.0 is 100 time more acidic than 7.0. And, pH 4.0 is 1000 times more acidic than 7.0.

The same holds for alkaline or base pH values above pH 7.0 but unlike acids, which as the pH goes down the acid strength goes up, alkaline pH increase in strength as their value goes up. An alkaline solution of 8.0 is ten time stronger than solution of 7.0. See the chart below for more information on how pH strength changes from one value to the other.

A pH of 1 (Stomach Acid) 1,000,000 (H)+ atoms Acid
A pH of 2 (Lemon Juice) 100,000 (H)+ atoms Acid
A pH of 4 (Tomato Juice) 1,000 (H)+ atoms Acid
A pH of 6 (Saliva) 10 (H)+ atoms Acid
A pH of 7 (Water) 1 (H)+ atoms Neutral
A pH of 8 (Sea Water) 10 (H)+ atoms Alkaline
A pH of 10 (Milk of Magnesia) 1,000 (H)+ atoms Alkaline
A pH of 12 (Soapy Water) 100,000 (H)+ atoms Alkaline
A pH of 14 (Liquid Drain Cleaner) 10,000,000(H)+ atoms Alkaline

The basic unit of pH is the H+, hydrogen ion. pH is a measure of the amount of Hydrogen ions that exists in a solution. The more hydrogen ions that exist in a solution the more acidic it becomes and the more damaging it becomes to cells and tissue in your body.

Water is considered neutral. It is neither an acid nor alkaline and has a pH of 7.0. What this means is that water has as many H+ ions as OH-, hydroxyl ions. Water's chemical formula is H_2O, which is equal to two H+ and one OH-. When chemicals are mixed with water, the mixture can become either acidic or basic.

You don't need to understand the mathematics of this definition, but there it is. What is important is that you understand that a pH of 1.0 is very acidic and if you were to put your hand in it, it would damage your skin immediately. A pH of 12 is a highly alkaline solution and is not as damaging as acid, but it would still burn your skin.

A pH less than 7 is acidic and a pH greater than 7 is basic. When a liquid is an acid, we call it an acidic solution or an acid solution. When a liquid is a base we called it a basic solution or an alkaline solution. I will be using these terms interchangeably.

Acid forming Food – is food that when metabolized or digested by your cells leaves a residue or ash that is acidic. It is this acid that is released by your cells into your lymph liquid. This acid can then move into your tissues or be eliminated through the lymph node, move into your blood, then to the kidneys and out through your urine. Acid waste can also find its way into the colon for disposal.

Unfortunately, acid wastes, in the colon, that are not eliminated can be reabsorbed through the colon wall and into the liver and put back into general circulation. They then deposit in the tissue. It is the amount of acid residues left in your body that determine sickness or health.

Alkaline forming ash comes from the food you eat. This ash changes the pH in your cells and outside your cells to a less acidic liquid or an alkaline liquid. For good health and a clean body, you want to eat those foods that have alkaline ash, since these alkaline ions can neutralize acid wastes and prevent them from accumulating and causing damage in your body.

The determination of alkaline forming or acidic forming food is not what the pH of the food is before you eat it. An acid food before eating can be an alkaline forming food after it is metabolized by your cells. This concept can be a bit confusing, since you are not normally thinking about what your food becomes after it's used up by your cells. The left over, after your cell uses the food you eat always produces a residue that can be acidic or alkaline.

pH Of An Acid Body

Acid Body – you are considered to have an acid body if your overall body liquid pH is below 7.0. As your body changes to lower pH values the more susceptible you become for creating disease. Here's your sickness level vs. your pH level.

pH level of around 7.5 – healthy
pH level of 6.0 to 6.5 – not feeling good and are starting to create disease
pH level of 5.0 to 6.0 - has major health problems
pH level of 4.5 – 5.0 – have a terminal disease

pH of an Alkaline Body

Alkaline Body – you are considered to have an alkaline body, if your overall body liquid is a pH of 7.4. This is the pH level that you should strive for.

Here are 3 simple tests that you can do with your pH litmus paper.
These tests can give you an idea of how alkaline or acidic your body is and how strong your alkaline reserves are. Write down your reading and keep track of each test.

Saliva Test

Here is a simple test you can perform on your saliva that will give you an idea of where you stand with your body's pH level. Your saliva contains mineral salts that keep it alkaline at 7.4. If your body is deficient in alkaline food or minerals, it will take the minerals from your saliva causing it to drop in pH.

Keep in mind there are some inaccuracies with this method, since your body fluids are always in transition. This test simply gives you an idea of what your saliva pH is at that moment. Use this information for you own education. Then as you begin to change your eating habits and life style, you can retest to see if there is a difference.

Many doctors deny the accuracy or use of a saliva test and say it is of no value. Frankly, they prefer you to pay them a visit so that they can put you under their care, but, in an article written by Dr. Steven Zodkoy, *A Free and Simple Test for pH, a Potential Health Tester*, he promotes the use of this test.

URL: http://ezinearticles.com/?A-Free-and-Simple-Test-for-pH,-a-Potential-Health-Tester&id=2928

Another important issue related to pH is oxygen level. Tissue and cells have more oxygen available to them, when your body pH is 7.4 as compared to when it is 6.4.

It has been found that the average American's tissue pH is between 5.5 and 6.0. This indicates that they have a severe lack of oxygen in their cells and lymph liquid. Lack of oxygen in the body is known to create serious terminal diseases.

Those of you with acid bodies and that lack cell and lymph oxygen can correct your condition by learning what it takes to bring your body back to an alkaline level. This will give your body a chance to repair tissue and organs, provided they have not been severely damaged.

By testing your pH regularly, you can decide the validity of using pH litmus paper to determine the level of your health. As you make changes, you can test your saliva or urine to see, if color changes occur.

You need to take this test for 3 days and at least 3 times a day and get an average value so that you can establish a base line or a starting point for yourself.

Purchase some pH litmus paper at a drug store, laboratory outlet or order it through the internet. But, buy litmus paper that changes in increments of .25, .20, or small

Saliva pH Test

Gather saliva in your mouth then swallow. Do this three times. Place the pH paper under your tongue to wet it and then remove it. Let it sit for less than a minute and record the pH. Or, you can spit on it, then check for a color change.

Do this test around 1 hour before eating or around 2 hours after eating.

Saliva and Lemon Test

Do this test immediately after you do the saliva test above. Squeeze half of lemon juice in one ounce of water and swish it around in your mouth for 5 seconds or so then spit it out.

Wait one minute.

Now, measure your mouth's pH with litmus paper. Just place the paper into your mouth and wet it.

Now compare the color and pH value of this reading with your first pH saliva reading. This reading should have a higher alkaline reading than your first saliva reading.

If this reading has a higher alkaline reading, it means you have alkaline reserves. The higher the alkaline reading the have stronger your alkaline reserves. A smaller alkaline upward change means you have alkaline reserves, but they are not as strong as they should be.

If your pH reading does not change from your first reading or actually goes down by becoming more acidic, then your alkaline reserves are weak and you need to make some major changes in the way you eat. In this book, I will show you what you will need to do to bring up your alkaline reserves, so that you will not be susceptible to serious diseases.

Urine pH test

There have been clinical studies indicating that urine pH is an accurate reflection of your body responds to the production acid waste. Each time you test your urine in the morning, note what you eat in your evening meal. Eating a high protein meal, which is an acid meal, will require more alkaline ash to neutralize your acid dinner. If you eat a meal high in vegetables and little protein then your body should easily neutralize your meal by morning.

Here's how to do the urine pH test.

In the morning when you urinate, allow it to flow for a second and then wet your pH litmus paper with urine.

If your urine pH is below 6.4 this indicates that your body did not have enough alkaline ash or ions to neutralize your previous evening dinner. In addition, you do not have enough alkaline mineral reserves to protect your body from acid damage to your cells and tissues.

Your morning urine should be between 6.4 and 7.4, indicating that your alkaline reserves are in good shape. The closer to 7.4 is better.

If your morning urine is over 7.4 and higher, this indicates your body is going into an emergency state, using ammonia from your liver in an effort to reduce your acid body. You may read as high as 8.0 indicating for sure you are producing ammonia to neutralize your acid dinner. To change this will require a substantial change in your eating habits.

Test you urine for 7 days to see if it remains consistent.

Record this information to see how it changes as you progress and change your eating habits during the next 30 days.

Use these tests to make adjustments in your eating habits. By eating more fruits and vegetables throughout the day and for sure in the evening, you will make your body more alkaline. You can test for this and prove it to yourself.

Chapter 3: Vegetables That Give You The Best Health

Vegetables to eat

The best way to maintain better health is to eat more fruits and vegetables. Vegetable have a high level of nutrition provided they are organic, are eaten raw, have very little cooking, and are eaten soon after harvest.

The purpose of eating more produce is to get best possible nutrition, and to detoxify and maintain your body in an alkaline condition. Vegetable are high in most of the vitamins, minerals, antioxidants, and nutrients that you need for good life.

What vegetables do is bring more oxygen into your body and all organs. It makes your body alkaline. It is well known now that when your body fluids are acidic, you will be prone to more illness and disease. First of all, acid in your body creates inflammation. Low grade inflammation that you don't feel, slowly leads to the deterioration of organs and tissue. That is why as your years pass, you start to see the appearance of various diseases in your body.

Second, there are various pathogens that like an acid environment and setup household in your body. As these pathogens, bacteria, viruses, and parasite multiple, they make your body more acidic because of their excretions.

Here is the list of vegetables to eat in order of priority. All of these vegetable will neutralize your body acid, since they contain minerals that are acid binding. Those vegetables that are from 50% to 100% Acid Binding will eliminate acids from your body. Those vegetables that are closer to 100% will eliminate more acids from your body. But eating all of these vegetable will give you great health benefits.

Vegetables at 93% Acid Binding – best vegetables to eat
Kelp, Seaweed, Watercress, Asparagus

Vegetables at 80% Acid Binding – Still the best to eat
Lettuce Leaf, Oyster plant, Pumpkin, Spinach, Squash, Peas, Carrots, Celery, Chard, Swiss, Dandelion greens

Vegetables at 73% Acid Binding – Great vegetables to eat
Bamboo shoots, Beets, Broccoli, Cabbage, Cauliflower, Collards, Corn, sweet, Ginger (fresh), Mushrooms, Mustard greens, Onions, Pepper, Potatoes, Green, Lima, String, Potatoes

Vegetables at 67% Acid Binding – eat plenty of these
Brussell sprouts, Cucumbers, Eggplant, Okra, Onions, Radishes, Tomatoes

Vegetable juices at 80% to 93% Acid Binding
Parsley, wheat grass, carrot, celery (see the juice chapter for more juices to drink)

Soy Bean Products at 60% Acid Binding – Limit your use of tofu since it is a genetically modified organism, GMO
Dried beans, Soy cheese, Soy milk, Tempeh, Tofu

Here is additional information on vegetables you should be eating.

Broccoli

Broccoli is a woman's favorite vegetable to eat and for good reason. It is rich in chlorophyll which absorbs heavy metal and detoxifies the body. It is capable of blocking cell mutations, which gives it its anti-cancer properties. Its rich in minerals and vitamins that help your body become more alkaline. It stimulates the liver to produce enzymes that destroy carcinogens. Broccoli can reduce your risk of stomach, oral cavity, lung, pharynx, prostate, esophageal, and colon cancer.

It has helped in obesity, blood toxicity, neuritis, and high blood pressure; use it at least three times a week. It has been known to relieve the symptoms of migraine headaches.

Brussels Sprouts

Brussels sprouts are similar to cabbage. They contain the phytochemicals sulforaphane, indole-3-carbinol, dithiolethione, and isotheocynates. They also have anticancer protease inhibitors – beta-carotene and vitamin A. You can use them for catarrh, acid body, constipation, hardening of the arteries, and bleeding gums.

Cabbage

Cabbage is an important vegetable, since it has so many curative activities in your body. It has been used to cure every known disease that man has acquired. It is one of the oldest vegetable to be cultivated. It has been used to cure yeast infections that occur anywhere on your body. It has been show to inhibit tumor growth in the colon and rectum. It can lower LDL, bad cholesterol and raise your good cholesterol, HDL.

It contains so called "phase II enzymes", which inactivates major carcinogens by destroying their molecular centers. In addition, over 100 glucosinolates have been identified in the Brassica family (cabbage, Brussels sprouts, cauliflowers, and broccoli). These glucosinolates can inhibit the growth of cancer cells and they are antibacterial and anti-fungal.

Cabbage is recommend for building muscles, blood cleansing and eye strengthening. It is also good for teeth, gums, hair, nails, bones, asthma, gout, constipation, diabetes, and skin. It also has a history of providing relief for ulcers, whether eaten raw, cooked, or as juice.

You should be eating cabbage every day, either raw or cooked.

Carrots

Carrots are another super food because of its high vitamin A. You will get health benefits from the vegetable, whether you use it raw or as a juice.

Carrots in the past have been used to cure stomach aches and as aphrodisiac. Since they are high in beta-carotene, they are useful in eye conditions and in preventing and fighting cancer. Beta carotene is converted to vitamin A in the liver.

Carrots have also been used for purifying the blood, constipation, asthma, poor complexion, poor teeth, insomnia, inflamed kidney and bladder, colitis, hair and nails.

Cauliflower

Cauliflower has high vitamin A content. It serves as a good blood purifier and has some use in asthma, kidney and bladder disorders, high blood pressure, gout, poor complexion, and constipation. Eat the leaves for their mineral content.

Cauliflower can cause indigestion and poor food assimilation and should be used in moderation.

Celery

Celery is high in sodium. This sodium is called organic sodium as compared with inorganic sodium which comes from table salt. Organic sodium does not cause problems in the body, because it has the right energy associated with it and the body knows how to use it. The stomach is called a sodium organ, because it uses so much sodium in its lining to prevent your stomach acid from creating an ulcer.

Sodium is also used in your lymph liquid, which surrounds your cells. It acts as an electrolyte and is in ion form moving in and out of your cell structure to maintain a certain potential or voltage across your cell membrane. This voltage must be maintained so that other nutrients can go into the cell and so toxic matter can come out. Keeping this voltage, by eating vegetables, within a specific range is what gives you excellent health. For this reason you should be including those vegetables that contain plenty of sodium.

Celery is useful in diseases of the kidney, arthritis, rheumatism, neuritis, constipation, high blood pressure, asthma, excess mucus, and diabetes. Celery is also good for an over worked brain, gallstones, teeth, anemia, and insomnia

Chard

Chard is high in potassium, sodium, and calcium. These are all organic minerals that create an alkaline body. In raw form chard contains oxalic acid, but when cooked, it has more oxalic acid. It is best to eat chard raw. Cooked chard creates higher levels of oxalate, which can form crystal that can deposit in your stomach and kidneys. These crystals can be quite painful.

In addition, oxalic acid combines with calcium to form calcium oxalate, which is the chemical composition of kidney stones.

Eating raw chard provides the body with a little organic oxalic acid, which plays an important part in maintaining the elimination organs. Chard keeps these organs in good tone and helps create stimulating peristaltic action in the gastrointestinal tract.

Taking calcium supplements, when you eat vegetables high in oxalic acid, will cause calcium oxalate to form in your stomach. This action stops calcium from getting into your blood stream. In general, most people can process and eliminate oxalic acid. There are some people who by genetics are not able to process oxalic acid and are prone to oxalate crystal.

Chard is useful for anemia, constipation mucus accumulation, obesity, and poor appetite.

You can add young chard to your salads, since the mature chard leaves are bitter. If you want to cook them, do it in a little water for 10-15 minutes, under low heat.

Chick Peas

Chick peas are also known as garbanzo beans. They are extremely high in protein and at the same time high in potassium, which is good for the heart. It has cholesterol-reducing phytosterols and iron and calcium to build your bones. This bean is quite good for B vitamins, such as niacin, thiamine, and riboflavin.

Collards

This green leafy vegetable is high in alkaline minerals. It is a great vegetable if you have an acid body, anemia, liver problems, and arthritis. If you are trying to get off drugs, use collards.

Cucumber

Cucumbers are one of the best natural diuretic, which promotes the flow of urine. This makes it useful for both high and low blood pressure. It also has the enzyme "erepsin", which helps digest protein.

Its high silicon and sulfur content helps promote hair and nail growth and it is good for teeth and gum health.

Cucumber is widely used in salads, but some recipes call for cucumbers in soups.

Garlic

Garlic is another super food. It is beneficial in all kinds of body conditions and ailments. It should be used daily in all the different cooking you do. It is one of the best foods for your digestive and lymph system. It is used to help eliminate toxic matter from your body and to help clean your blood.

It is good for your cardiovascular system and for activating peristaltic action. It has been found to be good for colds, asthma, catarrh, fevers, gas, bronchitis, thyroid hypo-function sinusitis, and for the release of phlegm and mucus.

Horseradish

Horseradish helps to remove excess mucus from your body, including your nasal and sinus cavities. It is used for colds, coughs, and asthma. It can be used to stimulate your appetite. It can be irritating to your kidneys and bladder. Use only 1/4 of a teaspoon at a time. Mixing with equal amounts lemon juice, you can take this 4 times a day.

Hot Chili Peppers

Hot chili peppers have a substance called capsaicin, which makes chili peppers hot. This substance has the ability to block pain messages that travel on the nerve network. Pain is transmitted along nerves by a chemical called Substance P. Capsaicin has the ability to reduce substance P and thereby reducing pain transmissions.

Lentils

Lentils are another nutritious food, which are rich in protein, fiber, alkaline and acid minerals. Lentils are anti-toxic and are used for treating anemia, dyspepsia, and intestinal inflammation.

Mung Bean Sprouts

Mung Bean Sprouts are great for malnutrition. They are capable of eliminating toxic matter from your body and provide some restoration effects. Sprouts have a high level of active minerals and this make them a power food. Mung sprouts have been found to be good for arthritis, neuritis, constipation, and other common illnesses.

Mustard green

Mustard greens are very high in potassium. Use it for an overall body tonic. It helps in anemia, constipation, rheumatism, arthritis, body acid, kidney and bladder ailments, and bronchitis. Pregnant and nursing mothers should eat mustard greens for their mineral and vitamin content.

Use mustard greens in your salad or sandwiches. They can also be blended with fruit juices in a blender. You can add them to your soups. You can also cook them in water for 10 minutes, under low heat. Keep them covered, while cooking, to minimize the loss of liquid.

Onion

Onions are high in potassium and are capable of neutralizing body acids. They help increase the flow of urine and have a slight laxative effect. They also have an antiseptic property. They help drain mucus and loosen phlegm. Onions are good for hair, nails and eyes. They are useful for asthma, bronchitis, pneumonia, influenza, and colds.

Onions have been found helpful in tuberculosis, low blood pressure, insomnia, neuritis, vertigo, obesity, and worm and parasite elimination. You can use them as a poultice on your chest for inflammation of your lungs or for boils on your skin. Use onion in all of your cooking.

Okra

Okra has some protein but not all the amino acids and provides sodium and calcium. Okra is good for reducing the inflammation of the stomach and intestines created by ulcers. It is also good for lung inflammation and colitis. It is good for sore throat and weight loss when use frequently.

Potato, Sweet

This potato is great when you are doing heavy work as it has plenty of minerals and vitamins. It is used for ulcers and inflamed colon. If you have low blood pressure because of poor blood circulation, eat sweet potatoes. These potatoes are good, if you have hemorrhoids or diarrhea

Pumpkin

Pumpkin is a winter squash and has more nutrients than the summer squash. It can be used in burns where you have intense pain. This is accomplished by putting a can of pumpkin or cooked pumpkin in the refrigerator overnight then covering the burn with cold mashed pumpkin.

There is also some evidence that eating pumpkin and yellow vegetables lowers your risk of creating cancer, especially lung cancer. You can use pumpkin seeds to get rid of parasites or tape worms by chewing on a cup of pumpkin seeds every day for about 5 days.

Because pumpkins are high in vitamin A, they can be used for people who need to strengthen they eye sight. They are good for eliminating fluids in body cavities, infected or inflamed intestines, stomach ulcers, hemorrhoids, and high blood pressure.

Most pumpkin is used for pies and cookies. There are other deserts that can be made with pumpkin, including pumpkin custard.

Parsley

Parsley is seldom used as a vegetable to eat, since it is mostly used as garnish. But you can add it to your salads and to your soups. It is one vegetable that is high in fat soluble chlorophyll.

The chlorophyll obtained from green vegetables is more nutritious and has more curative properties than the liquid chlorophyll you purchase in a health store. The store chlorophyll is water soluble and is not utilized as good as fat soluble chlorophyll.

Parsley's high mineral and vitamin content makes it valuable for anemia, inflamed kidneys, tuberculosis, halitosis, menstruation disorders, fevers, congested liver and gall bladder issues, urinary tract diseases, obesity, high blood pressure, mucus release and venereal disease.

Always eat parsley raw. You can add it to your soup when you are ready to serve it. As a tea, it has been found useful for diabetics. For people recovering from illness, a broth of chopped parsley, tomatoes, and potatoes skins served with raw milk and real butter provides nutrition for recovering.

Radishes

Radishes are part of the cabbage family. They are high in vitamin C and potassium. Potassium helps in making your body more alkaline. Radishes have a beneficial effect on teeth, gums, nerves, hair, and nails. They stimulate appetite and relive nervous exhaustion. They help to relieve constipation and mucus flow. They are useful for obesity, liver disorders, and will help to dissolve gallstones. They also have a slight diuretic effect.

Radishes can be eaten raw or can be cooked. To cook, cover them with water and cook for 15 – 20 minutes. Cooking water can be used as a drink to get the benefit of the mineral that leach out.

Spinach

Spinach has been found helpful for anemia, constipation neuritis, nerve exhaustion, tumors, insomnia, arthritis, obesity high blood pressure, bronchitis, and indigestion. It also is used for kidney, bladder and liver problems. It has a high iron content that is useful in anemia. It also contains Choline and Inositol, which helps prevent arteriosclerosis.

Sprouts

Sprouting seeds, legumes, and whole grains are the healthiest thing you can do. Once a seed is sprouted, it contains vitamins, minerals, and enzymes. Sprouts will help to make your body more alkaline. They are easy to digest since they are living food.

You can easily grow your own sprouts. If you decide to do this, start with alfalfa seeds. But you can sprout lentils, mung beans, rye, soy, wheat, sunflower, and radish seeds.

Turnip and Turnip Greens

Turnip roots are useful in eliminating constipation and tuberculosis. They also can relieve nervousness and insomnia. When eaten raw, they are good for teeth and gums. You can boil turnips and use the water to relieve coughs, throat hoarseness and asthma.

Turnips can be eaten raw in salads or cut up and boiled for 20 minutes in a small amount of water. They can also be added to soups.

Turnip greens – are high in vitamins and minerals, which can reduce the amount of acid in your body. Because of this, they offer relief for a variety of different body conditions – anemia, poor appetite, tuberculosis, obesity, high blood pressure, bronchitis, asthma, liver ailments, gout, and bladder disorders. They are also good for your complexion, for blood purification, and for eliminating bacterial toxins from the blood.

Cut up these greens in small pieces and cooked them for 20 – 30 minutes in the smallest amount of water. Doing this will preserve the high potassium and calcium that they have, which will help you get rid of body acids.

Tomato

Tomato is actually a fruit, but most people think of it as vegetable. Tomatoes have a natural antiseptic property and protect against infections. They improve skin and purify the blood. Tomatoes help in cases of gout, rheumatism, tuberculosis, high blood pressure and sinus problems. It is useful in liver congestion and in dissolving gallstones. The nicotinic acid in tomatoes helps reduce cholesterol and the vitamin K helps prevent hemorrhaging. Because of the high lycopene, they serve as a strong antioxidant.

Tomatoes can be prepared in a number of ways and still provide the nutritional value that they have. They can be baked, broiled, canned.

Watercress

Watercress has been used for eye disorder, excess weight, arthritis, rheumatism, bleeding gums and hardening of the arteries. It is also useful in kidney and liver disorders. Use watercress whole or finely chopped up in salads. You can use watercress as an ingredient in other recipes. Or when you prepare vegetable juices, you can add it to a blender when mixing your juices.

Many of the vegetables have over lapping benefits, but they all have one specific illness that they benefit more than any other vegetable. Vegetables, fruits, and herbs are where pharmaceuticals look to find new chemicals that they can use to create drugs. But vegetables are a complete food and they have the all the nutrients balanced. When you eat them, they provide the nutrients your body needs in a way that your body can use them.

Vegetables and fruits can heal and cure your illness; you just need to know which ones to use and then use them in larger quantities then you normally do.

CHAPTER 4: ALKALINE VEGETABLE JUICE TO DRINK

Vegetable Juices

Try to use those vegetables that you typically don't use. These vegetables will help you detoxify more. Stay away from the iceberg lettuce, since it has little nutritional value and is hard to digest. You can use romaine and butter lettuce, but try to use some of the other dark green leafy ones.

Dark green lettuce, Beets, Carrots, Cucumbers, Cabbage, Tomatoes, Parsley, Onions, Spinach, Turnips, Asparagus, Garlic

Fresh vegetable juices have high nutritional, healing, and curing powers. Using vegetable juices as juice therapy has been used throughout the world and for centuries to help the body recover from nearly every body aliment. By separating the juice from its fiber, its minerals and nutrients are suspended in the distilled water of the juice. This allow for your body to digest and absorb vegetable juices within minutes as compared to hours when eating the entire vegetable.

Consider vegetable drinks as a meal. You should not drink them with your meals or with any other food. You can add brewer's yeast, vitamin C powder, or acidophilus powder to them. You can take digestive enzymes with those juices that are not fresh and that come in a can, bottle, or are frozen.

Avoid those packaged vegetable juices that are high in salt content. If you are drinking tomato juice, drink only the juice that is 100% tomato.

You can mix certain juices together to get a better taste. You can use the pulp from juicing vegetables to thicken soups or for a compost pile.

If you don't like to eat vegetables or if you are sick and need to recover, then juicing is the ideal way to get nutrients into your body. Juicing vegetables is another way to get the benefits of vegetables without eating them. Juicing them does not get you the entire benefit of the whole vegetable.

Carrot Juice

Carrot juice is the king of juices, since it has so many health benefits and can be mixed with other juices to make them more palatable. It rejuvenates the body, produces fresh blood, cleanses the body, produces glowing skin, and provides nutrients for healthy eyes and liver. For those that have health issue, carrot juice daily is a must to help bring the body back to health.

Its juice helps you maintain the proper balance between alkaline and acid body. Because of it high vitamin A and E, carrot juice is effective in promoting bones and teeth and most importantly the maintenance of healthy body tissues and glandular function.

It also has vitamin B, C, D, and K. Pregnant women should include carrot juice in their diet and during nursing for their health and for the health of their baby. If you have a low white blood count then carrot juice can bring it up.

You can take carrot juice indefinitely and in any reasonable quantity – 1 to 4 pints a day is ok. If you have digestion or appetite problems, carrot juice is must. If you need help in keeping your teeth healthy, carrot juice will help improve your jaw and teeth structure.

In his book, N.W. Walker, Doctor of Science, Water Can Undermine Your Health, Prescott, Norwalk Press, 1974, recounts his experience with carrot juice,

"There was a time, when I first started drinking carrot juice that my skin took on an orange yellow hue. I discovered that this was due to the cleansing of my liver, which happened to be in VERY bad condition at the time. However, after a few months the discoloration disappeared and my skin was better and clearer than it had ever been."

If you decide to drink carrot juice daily, there could be a time when you start to feel sick or distressed. Most likely it's not a result of drinking too much carrot juice but more that you have a lot of body toxins to get rid of.

Carrot juice is great for improving your eyesight. If you need to pass an eye sight test and are worried you might not, drink a few glasses of carrot juice daily, for a few weeks and then take your test.

If you have ulcers, then juice cabbage, this juice will help to heal them. But combine cabbage juice with carrot juice. If you have cancer, then drinking carrot juice can be helpful in nourishing these cells back to normal in combination with other therapies. With cancer you would need to take a lot of carrot juice daily.

Celery Juice

Celery Juice has a high level of potassium, and if you need potassium, then this is the juice to drink. You can add carrot juice to this juice to make it more palatable. Celery juice is also high in sodium and is considered a sodium food. Your stomach is considered a sodium organ, because it needs a lot of sodium to protect its walls from your stomach acid.

If you frequently feel nervous or agitated, try drinking a combination of celery and carrot juice. This combination is good for restoring the function of degenerating nerve sheathing.

In the case, where you feel like you have an acid body, then celery juice is a must. Combining it with carrot juice will definitely move you toward a more alkaline body.

The sodium in celery is organic and has nothing to do with the effects of table salt, which has inorganic sodium that the body cannot use. You cannot overdose with natural organic sodium, since the body will eliminate the excess organic sodium in your body. However, when you eat table salt, you can overdose with this sodium. When you do overdose, the kidney has to find a place to store this sodium or eliminate it from your body. When this sodium is stored, it leads to edema and high blood pressure, because of the water the sodium attracts.

Use celery juice, if you have allergies, blood poisoning from an intensive burn, stepping on an old nail, or having a urinary infection.

Cucumber Juice

You can use cucumber juice to mix with other juices, when you do not have carrot juice. Cucumber juice is a great source of manganese and is high in vitamin A. If you have a low blood count then this is the juice for you. Cucumber juice is one of the best diuretics you can use when you need to promote urine.

Because of its high silicon and sulfur levels, it is good for hair and nail growth. Carrot juice, celery, and cucumber juice are good for rheumatic conditions. With its high potassium content, it is good for high and low blood pressure. This juice has also been found to be helpful in skin eruptions.

Dandelion Juice

This juice is high in those minerals that neutralize acids in your body, so use it, if you have an acid body. It is one of the richest foods in magnesium and iron. With all the minerals, found in this plant, your teeth will benefit with strength and firmness.

Garlic Onion Juice

Garlic belongs to the onion family. It is recommended not juicing garlic, since you can get the liquid form in two ounce bottle from Kyolic. When juicing onion, try to find the Vidalia or Walla Walla onions, since they are sweeter. Combine these juices with other juices such as parsley, watercress, or spinach. For 1/4 cup of onion juice, put 1 teaspoon of garlic. Start slow with the use of these juices and experiment with the quantity until you get use to their tastes.

The combination of onion and garlic provide many complex compounds, but they have 3 important minerals – sulfur, potassium and germanium.

In his book, Heinerman, John, Heinerman's Encyclopedia of

Healing Juices, Parker Publishing Company, New York,1994, says it all about garlic and onion,

"The final and most important mineral in garlic and onions is sulphur. Doctors, nutritionists, and health writers don't seem to give much attention to this particular trace element.

I've spent almost a decade studying this tremendously important mineral and have discover in all of the research surveyed (including my own) that it is the key to preventing hardening of the arteries, cholesterol buildup in the heart, and for stopping drug-resistant forms of bacteria and fungus.

When combined with other elements such as potassium and germanium in spices like garlic and onion, a powerful trio of chelating agents are formed which keep the heart and liver free of fatty deposits, the immune defenses alert and active, and the condition of the skin healthy and young."

Garlic and onion juice are also effective for encephalitis, an infection of herpes simplex virus, and for meningitis virus, or other viruses. This juice will also eliminate intestinal parasites in the stomach, small intestine and colon.

Green Pepper Juice

There are many different green peppers, some are not hot and some will burn your mouth – bell peppers, habanero, jalapeno, pimento, and Tabasco sauce.

The bell pepper juice is high in silicon, which is what your hair and nails need. It is also useful for your tear-ducts and sebaceous glands. In combination with carrot juice, this drink is great for clearing up skin blemishes. Use around 1/4 green pepper juice to 3/4 carrot juice.

Hot chilies have been found to assist in holding back the progression HIV/Aids. One Chile that some people have experimented with is the Korean spicy pickled cabbage called KIM-CHI, which has a lot of cayenne pepper. The compounds in this and other hot chilies appear to increase the production of killer T-cells, interleukin-2, and other power immune factors.

It has been found that countries, like Thailand and Mexico, have lower incidents of thrombosis, clots in blood vessels. This may be due to the capsaicin in the peppers they frequently eat.

Green Juices

Green drinks can help your pancreas to control blood sugar levels through the production of insulin. It does this by rebuilding the pancreas so that glucagon and insulin are created throughout the day. A green drink can be used every day. Try to use a green drink at least twice a week.

Using liquid chlorophyll is great, if you don't have a green drink. Squeeze the juice of one lemon into 1/2 oz. of chlorophyll then add 6 oz. of water. You can drink this every day, first thing in the morning. You can use any amount of liquid chlorophyll you want, but add to it lemon juice or other juices to make it more drinkable. You can get liquid chlorophyll at your health food store.

Blue Green Manna is another powder you can use. It is high in chlorophyll and enzymes. This Manna is great for regulating the pancreas. You can check out this site for capsules. You can add a couple of ounces of fresh pineapple, apple, and grape juice to make it more palatable. Adding a pinch of honey is another way to take a green drink.

For kids you can add the green drink or green manna into jello.

In his book, Dr. Beddoe, A.F., Biologic Ionization as applied to Human Nutrition, S & J Unlimited, Washington, 1994, gives you a recipe for a fresh green drink that you can prepare with a blender,

"Take 2 cups of your favorite juice and place it in a good quality high speed blender. Add to it this large handfuls of greens chosen from the list that follows this paragraph. The amount will vary according to the type of blender used. . . Add as much as can be chopped and blended thoroughly and comfortably, until all greens have well blended for a period of time (3 to 4 minutes) turn off the blender and pour the mixture through a kitchen strainer to remove the pulp. The juice that is left is the green drink."

Use any of the following green leaves to create a green drink: dandelion, nasturtium leaves, parsley, wheat grass, pea pods, romaine lettuce, spinach, beet tops, carrot tops, celery stalk tops, kale, or any other dark green leaves.

The more chlorophyll you can drink and get into your body the better. Chlorophyll is one of the compounds that green drinks give you. Chlorophyll will slowly chelate, tie up and remove toxic heavy metals out of your body. It gives you great antibacterial and antiviral protection. And, it gives you good oxygenation for your cells. It is one of the best blood cleansers and rejuvenators, and it does this by building up your blood.

All dark green lettuce leaves are also high in iron and magnesium. Iron is constantly being used by your body to create blood hemoglobin. Any time blood is lost, your body has to create replacement blood and needs iron to do this. Your liver and the spleen are storage areas for iron and are ready to move your iron when new blood is needed. If you are iron deficient, then you need to use green drinks every day.

Horseradish Juice

Horseradish is a member of the mustard family and is a large root, which is grounded up to dress meat. It has a strong, pungent flavor. It is very high in sulfur and potassium with average amounts of sodium, calcium and phosphorus.

This juice has been used in the past for hypothermia, where one suffers from a decrease in body temperature. It was use at 1/4 teaspoon three times a day between meals with apple cider vinegar and some salt.

With one tablespoon of horseradish juice to one tablespoon of hydrogen peroxide, you can detoxify the body of toxic chemicals. It is also used for mucus congestion in the chest or head. Use 3 tablespoons of this juice flavored with pure maple syrup.

Kale and Collard Juices

Kale is very high in alkaline minerals like calcium. You can mix kale juice with carrot or pineapple juice. Drinking kale or collard juices will help you absorb more calcium than when you drink milk. If you have osteoporosis, then you need the calcium provided by these juices.

Mustard Greens Juice

Pure mustard greens juice has an irritating effect to the

gastrointestinal tract and kidney. By combining this juice with carrot, spinach and turnip juice, you will get relief for your hemorrhoids.

Mustard greens have a high level of oxalic acid and should never be eaten cooked. When cooked, the oxalic acid is turned from organic oxalic acid, a natural nutrient your body can use, to an inorganic oxalic acid that your body cannot use.

Inorganic oxalic acid is destructive in your body, since it causes the formation of kidney oxalic crystal – kidney stones. Organic oxalic acid is an important nutrient that maintains the health of the gastrointestinal tract. It keeps it healthy, so that it can perform peristaltic action when it is needed.

Okra Juice

Okra juice has properties that help maintain your blood plasma levels despite losing blood during surgery or other types of conditions of blood loss. It has been used to alleviate the pain, muscle weakness, and fatigue that are common with autoimmune diseases.

Parsley Juice

Parsley juice should never be taken alone, but a small amount, one to two oz., should be mixed with other vegetable juices like carrot and Spinach. You can also mix it with lime and orange juice to get a different taste. It helps in keeping your blood vessels functioning normal. It has a tonic effect on the urinary system by removing urinary problems like bladder pain and swelling. It is also useful in kidney diseases.

Parsley juice is also good for the eyes. Use it with other juices as mentioned and it will help reduce corneal opacity, corneal ulceration, cataract, pupil haziness, and ophthalmia – inflammation of the eye, conjunctivitis, and weak vision.

It is also useful in relieving cramps associated with menstrual irregularities. But it has to be used a little more concentrated with the above juices mentioned.

Parsnip Juice

Parsnip juice is low in calcium and sodium, but because it is high in potassium phosphorus, sulfur, silicon and chlorine it is useful for lung and bronchial conditions. If you have pneumonia or emphysema then this is the juice to drink. Use only cultivated parsnip for juices; the wild parsnip contains some poisonous compounds. This juice is also good for brittle nails.

Parsnip juice has been used to breakup small kidney stones. Here's how to use it. Use 1/4 juice with 3/4 parts liquid chlorophyll and drink every day until you get rid of the stones.

You can also use parsnip juice to control your overeating cravings and this will help you lose weight.

Peppermint Juice

Peppermint is used in many medicines and salads. Its use has been as an additive in salads, desserts, candy, and chewing gum. It is use in balms as menthol. Its curative powers lie in stomach discomforts, since it helps digestion, removes flatulence, abdominal pain, and improve bowel function.

Its juice is more difficult to use, since only a small amount is needed to produce results. Start by squeezing out a small amount of this juice from the leaves and stem. Then, add it to water with a small amount of lemon juice to gargle or for bad breath. One of the best ways to use peppermint is as a tea. In this form, you can get the benefits of its juices and oils to quiet any digestive problems you might have.

Potato Juice

The combination of eating meat and cooked potatoes has the effect of intensifying the solanine poison, an alkaloid, of the potato. Green potatoes have a higher concentration of this poison.

The juice of potatoes is quite digestible and has proven to be helpful in clearing up skin blemishes. Combine it with carrot juice to get a better tasting juice.

This juice can also be used for gallstones. Use both, raw potato juice and cooked potato peeling broth, for a week two times a day. Use the juice and broth at different time of the day. You can add some flavoring to the broth, so it is more palatable.

If you have stomach problems, sensitive nerves, gout, or sciatica, then combine this juice with carrots, beet, and cucumber juice.

Radish Juice

At least 1/3 of radish content is potassium and 1/3 is sodium. The radish is also high in iron and magnesium. Potassium is necessary for good heart function and for maintaining muscle strength.

Radish juice has a pungent taste and should never be drunk alone. It is best to mix it with carrots, tomatoes, or lemon juices or a combination of all three. It's used in killing germs and removing toxins from the body. It is a great blood purifier and builder and helps blood circulation.

Radish juice is great for eye sight, as a nerve soother, and to eliminate intestinal worms. It is useful for removing kidney and gall-bladder stones. The juice can be used to massage into wrinkles to minimize them. It is also useful for rejuvenating and rebuilding muscles.

It has the ability to restore the tone of mucus membranes.
In Russian research, they discovered that the sulfur in red radishes was able to keep the production of the thyroid's thyroxine and calcitonin in balance. All that is needed is eating a few radishes a day or drinking a little radish juice mixed with other juices – carrot, tomato, or celery.

For constipation radish juice helps promote peristaltic action. And for a fatty liver or gallbladder inflammations, this juice can help break up the fat in the liver and reduce the gallbladder inflammation.

Rhubarb Juice

Rhubarb has a high concentration of oxalic acid and should not be eaten cooked. The inorganic oxalic acid, when eaten for a long time, causes crystals to deposit in various parts of the body, causing pain and discomfort.

It is best to avoid the use of rhubarb vegetable and juice, since many of its juice benefits can be obtained from other vegetables.

Romaine Lettuce Juice

Romaine juice is different from other green leaf juices. Its sodium content is 60% higher than its potassium content, whereas in other greens, potassium is higher. By adding some kelp juice to this juice, it has been found to be of value in strengthening the adrenal cortex function.

This makes this juice important in the treatment of Addison's disease where the adrenal glands are affected. But for this juice to have maximum impact, beets, celery, carrots, spinach, and Swiss chard must be added. Other fruits such as strawberries, tomatoes, figs, honey, and almonds also need to be used in Addison's treatment.

Spinach Juice

Spinach juice should be used by anyone with anemia, because of its high iron content. It is also useful in the entire gastrointestinal tract and especial useful for constipation and nervous disorders.

Because drug store laxatives work as irritants in the colon, your body will attempt to expel this irritant. The result is everything that is in the colon is expelled. Laxatives become addictive because every time you use a laxative, you need a large and larger irritation to move matter out of your colon. This is why natural laxative like spinach can help to normalize your bowel function and not become additive.

Spinach and Cabbage juice are good for neuralgia, a pain that runs along a damaged nerve. The pain may be recurring, sharp, and extreme just as in lower back pain.

Use Spinach juice as a general or nerve tonic. It is good for sterility, impotency, and fatigue. You can gargle with slightly warm spinach juice to get relief from a sore throat, tonsillitis, or cough. If you drink pure spinach juice in the morning, it will remove chronic constipation and toxic matter from the colon.

If you're pregnant, this juice will help you eliminate low iron deficiency. It will help you improve your and your baby's health. Spinach's iron is easily digested and gradually absorbed. Use it with other juices especially carrot.

Spinach is also high in organic oxalic acid and should not be eaten cooked. Eat it raw or juiced to get the natural oxalic acid that your body needs.

String Bean Juice

String bean juice and Brussels sprout juice have been found to improve the function of the pancreas. For these juices to be effective here is what is required. Combine the juice of carrot, lettuce, string beans, and Brussels sprouts and drink 2 pints per day and one pint of carrot and one pint of spinach juice. Use this regime until you see improvement in your pancreas function.

Tomato Juice

Tomato juice is to be used in raw form. It is a blood purifier and stimulates the blood circulation. It cleanses your body of toxins and is a worm killer. Tomatoes help keep your blood alkaline, reduce body acidity, resist diseases, cure liver and spleen disorders, and also remove chronic fever. Use tomato juice when you have a cold or flu. Those that have diabetes or prone to nervous conditions should drink tomato juice regularly.

For some people tomatoes juice can create irritation, cough,upset stomach, and kidney and urinary bladder stones. So, if you are prone to stones do not drink a lot of this juice.

Tomato juice contains lycopene, a potent antioxidant, which has been found to neutralize free radical damage at the cell level. Because of this activity, lycopene has shown to be effective in many types of cancer and cardiovascular diseases. Lycopene gives certain fruits and vegetables their red appearance. Lycopene is considered a carotenoid, but is not readily converted into vitamin A.

In cooked form, citric, malic, and oxalic acids become inorganic compounds and have a detrimental effect on your body.

It is best to drink raw tomato juice to get the best benefits from this juice. When raw juice is drunk with starches or sugar, it acts as an acid food, otherwise the body see it as an alkaline food.

Turnips Juice

Turnips are white or indigo and look like beet-root in shape. They belong to the family of radish, carrot, and beets. It has a mild sweet yet slight pungent taste and its juice is easy to digest.

Aside from its juice, Turnips can be eaten raw or steam cooked and it will still maintain its medicinal value. It is an excellent remedy for constipation, impacted bowels, poor liver function, and poor skin appearance. It can promote appetite and is an excellent digestive aid.

Turnip Juice aids in maintaining normal sugar metabolism. It is a diuretic and it helps promote strong bones. It is also used in gout, colds, asthma, and liver problems. Using its juice will help you maintain strong and healthy teeth.

Alfalfa Juice

Alfalfa has an array of great vitamins – A, C, K, and P – and over 21 trace and natural minerals. Of course, the actual intensity of the nutrient will depend on the soil it was grown in.

You can use alfalfa juice with any citrus or pineapple juice for allergies. The high alkaline minerals become active in your blood and neutralize any allergens that have activated your allergies.

Alfalfa has chemicals call saponins, which are detergent like compounds. It is these compounds that can scrub the internal surfaces of your arteries to remove plaque and to prevent its build up. Alfalfa helps you reduce the devastating effects of arteriosclerosis.

In cases where you have symptoms of an acid body, alfalfa is what you need. Gout is a result of acid compounds created by eating an excess of meat and not eating enough vegetables. Alfalfa with its high levels of alkaline minerals will eliminate gout.

Asparagus

This vegetable is very high the amino acid called asparagine and vitamin A. It is a good vegetable for the nucleic acids and substances call histones, which may be good for cancer prevention. Asparagus contain phytosterols that fight cancer and rutin that strengthens your arteries. Eating asparagus gives you the juice that is effective in breaking up oxalic acid crystals in the kidneys, and throughout your muscular system.

This juice makes it useful for those conditions that are related to oxalic acid crystals, such as neuritis, arthritis, gout, stones, and other inflammatory conditions. Just a few stems of this vegetable give you about 4-5% of your daily protein requirements.

Asparagus has an alkaloid call Asparagine in high amounts. Asparagine is a non-essential amino acid. Alkaloids are compounds mostly found in plants and some are good and some are poison. In this case, Asparagine is beneficial for the body. It is an alkaline food and it has been found that the nervous system needs it for proper functioning.

If you do not get it in food, your body will create it. The only way to get this alkaloid into your body is by drinking asparagus juice. When you cook asparagus, this nutrient is lost.

Pure asparagus juice is quite strong and you should mix it with carrot juice. This juice is used as a diuretic and is used for kidney dysfunctions. Its juice is capable of breaking up kidney oxalic stones. It has a history of curing patients with acute nephritis or Bright's disease, a severe kidney disease.

It is also good for regulating the prostate and for rheumatism. This juice is also good for people with anemia or who are convalescents.

Combining asparagus juice with beet, carrot, and cucumber juice can provide a variety of nutrients that will help you keep a healthier body.

This juice is good for cancer, eye disorders, gout, nervous conditions, or skin disorders.

Acne and eczema can also be help with this juice. If the acne or eczema is cause by an excess of acid in your body, then asparagus juice will help get rid of this acid, giving you an alkaline body. When this happens, acids will not be trying to come out through the skin and your skin issues will be eliminated.

Eat the tops of asparagus by cooking and juice the stems. When you drink the juice, your urine will have a different smell, which indicates your body is detoxifying.

Artichokes

This vegetable is a great source of silymarin with 6 mg. Sillymarin is an antioxidant and anticancer nutrient. Artichokes contain anticancer polyphenols and are a fair source of folic acid. It is also known for treating alcohol induced liver disease. Jerusalem Artichokes, not globe or French, can be used to replace potatoes and are good for people with diabetes.

Artichokes have powerful diuretic affect, which is helpful in stimulating the kidneys. It has been used effectively in dropsy. It has also been found effective in anemia, acid body, diarrhea, rheumatism, obesity, and neuritis. The artichokes are packed with potassium and have some calcium.

Artichoke, Jerusalem Juice

This juice is well known for controlling weight. It does this when this juice is used in a certain way. Artichokes have a high amount of inulin. This is not like insulin, but is a carbohydrate that moves quickly into your blood stream to provide energy for the liver, spleen and pancreas to help stabilize and normalize your sugar levels. This is a good juice for chronic fatigue syndrome, hypoglycemia, and diabetes.

Mix this juice with carrot juice in a one to one mixture.
Mix this juice with equal parts of carrot, alfalfa or beet juice. For a weight loss program, drink this juice through a straw and swish it around in your mouth before swallowing. This helps to reduce your cravings for sweet or junk food.

CHAPTER 5: FRUITS THAT CURE DISEASE

Eating Fruits

Fruits should be eaten raw and as fresh as possible. Within hours of fruits being picked, they lose around 10% or more of their nutritional value. They should not be peeled except for citrus fruits and non-organic fruits. The peel of a fruit is where most of the vitamins, minerals, and pectin are.

Fruits in markets that have been there a while are still a good source of nutrients, even though they have lost some of their nutritional value.

The best fruits come from the farmers market where the fruit has been picked the previous day or that day in the morning. Organic fruits can readily be eaten whole, but non-organic fruits need to be washed carefully to remove pesticides and preservatives.

Organic lemon peels can be eaten, but you need to develop a taste for the peel. In a smoothie it can be easier to take this taste.

Do not cut fruits until you are ready to eat them. They oxidize rapidly. You can see apples oxidize quickly, when cut open. Other fruits may not show the oxidizing process, like apples do, but they are also oxidizing.

For those of you that do office work or mental work, then a good fruit, fruit smoothie, and or fruit juice for breakfast will keep your mind sharp and fresh. This is the best type of breakfast to eat, since it is aligned with your body cycles (Body Cycles explained in another chapter).

There are some situations where you do want to eat a good solid meal in the morning. For those of you that do physical labor, a good morning breakfast of eggs and cereal will give you the calories you need for your strenuous, morning work.

Here are the fruits you should be eating:

Here is a list of the fruits that have the highest alkaline minerals and the ones that you should be eating to eliminate your body acids.

The percentage assigned to these fruits is based on fresh fruits that are organic and that they are not cooked, canned or mixed with sugar. If they are cook or otherwise processed in some fashion, this will reduce their effectiveness as an acid binding fruit. However, they will still be somewhat effective in acid binding.

Fruits above 50% in value are more acid binding, which means they will trap acid wastes better. The fruits that are at 50% at are neutral.

Here is the list of fruits to eat and drink in the order of priority.

1. Fruits at 100% Acid Binding – Best fruits To Eat And Drink Lemons, melons – any type, watermelon

2. Fruits at 93% Acid Binding – Great fruits To Eat And Drink Cantaloupes, dried dates, dried figs, limes, mango, papaya

3. Fruits at 87% Acid Binding – Still Great Fruits To Eat And Drink Kiwis, passion fruit, pineapples, raisins, umeboshi plums

4. Fruits at 80% Acid Binding – Eat And Drink These Fruits Apricots, avocados, bananas, fresh dates, fresh figs, currants, gooseberries grapes, grapefruits guavas, kumquats, nectarines, pears, persimmons, quince

5. Fruits at 73% Acid Binding – Still Fruits To Eat And Drink Apples, organs, peaches, pomegranate, raspberries, sour grapes, strawberries

6. Fruits at 67% Acid Binding – Still Neutralizes Acids, Eat And Drink This fruit

Citrus Fruits (See the section on citrus fruits in Fruit Juice chapter)

The citrus fruits are the fruits you should concentrate on eating. Eat them every day, if possible, fresh lemon juice in the morning in a warm glass of water and watermelon during the day.

Apples – eat 1 – 3 apples a day and eat at least one a day. Eat organic apples because you can eat the skins and most pectin is in the skin, which helps with constipation. Apples contain ascorbic acid, bioflavonoids, fiber, pectin, quercetin, minerals, and vitamins

Apples are high in soluble fiber, with the skin containing small amount of beta carotene. They contain vitamin C, potassium and some iron. Apples in the morning provide fiber and pectin, which helps to clean out your colon.

You can also eat dried apples, but most nutrients are lost in the drying process except iron and fiber.

Apricots – eat as many as you like. Apricots are a high source of minerals, fiber, and beta-carotene. (A precursor to vitamin A) They help to relieve or prevent constipation.

Apricots have a short season and that is why you see a lot of dried apricots for sale. Eat apricots in season.

Dried apricots are more nutritious than fresh, since the nutrients are more concentrated. The major problem with dried apricots is that they are dried with sulfur dioxide and this creates more acid and health issues for your stomach. There are some dried apricots that use low sulfur dioxide and some that use no sulfur dioxide. These are not as appealing as the sulfur dried ones.

Bananas – eat only one banana a day. Bananas have the phytochemicals fructoOligosaccharides, which feeds the good bacterial in your colon. By feeding the good bacteria, you prevent the bad bacteria from overtaking the colon and producing toxic acids that get into the skin.

Bananas are high in potassium and fiber. They are a good source of Folate, vitamin C, and B-6. Bananas contain practically no sodium. As you will see later, sodium is one of the top nutrients to consume. But only the sodium in fruits and vegetables is what your body needs.

Blackberries and blueberries – help cleanse the blood and are for hemorrhoids. They help a weak kidney and are good for creating good skin on your face.

Berries, blackberries, raspberries strawberries are all high in fiber and antioxidants. The deeper their colors – red, blue, and black - the more antioxidants they have. Antioxidants combine with free radicals in your body to deactivate them.

Cantaloupes – are high in vitamin A, C and have many other minerals. This makes them good for any type of skin problem. It is one the best fruits to eat. It has a high source of antioxidants, and beta carotene. It is also high in fiber.

Eat cantaloupe only with other melons and do eat it with other fruits. The stomach enzymes necessary to digest cantaloupes are different from other fruits and the stomach concentrates on digesting only similar types of fruit at a time.

Cherries – are good blood cleansers and help the liver and kidney. They are high in vitamin C, pectin, potassium and soluble fiber. Eating cherries and their juices will help you maintain regular bowel movement, when consumed between meals.

Figs - high in fiber and can be eaten fresh or dried. They are a good source of magnesium, potassium, calcium, iron, Vitamin B6 and Folate. Because they are high in sugar, their stickiness can contribute to tooth decay. So when you eat fresh fig rinse your mouth out with water afterwards.

Eating figs with other fruits high in Vitamin C will increase the absorption of iron.

Grapes – help cleanse the body, build blood, and build the body. They are good for constipation, skin, and liver disorders.

Grapes are high in pectin and bioflavonoids. They are a good source of iron, potassium and vitamin C. They provide for an excellent snack between meals. One problem with them is they are highly treated with pesticides.

Mango – is good for kidney inflammation. It contains a lot of minerals, which helps to neutralize acid waste.

Mangos are an excellent source of beta carotene, vitamin C and fiber. They contain vitamin E, niacin, potassium and iron. Mangos have been associated with a decrease in breast cancer with eaten regularly. Use it to make morning smoothies.

Strawberries – have been shown to have strong anti-acne activity. They are high in pectin content, which helps to keep your bowels moving.

Avocados – are a fruit. It is one of the fruits that is highest content of mono-unsaturated fatty acid, omega-9, which is a good fat. Most avocado fat consist of 60 - 75% omega-9. It also contains vitamin E, folic acid, fiber and many other nutrients. Omega-9 is an important omega to consume and not many foods contain this nutrient.

Papayas - contain the protein digestive enzyme papain. Papain is similar to pepsin, which is the digestive enzyme found in our stomach. They also contain a good amount of vitamin A, beta-carotene, potassium, and vitamin C.

As you can see many of the fruits contain a lot of vitamin C, potassium, sodium, beta carotene, antioxidants, bioflavonoids, minerals, and fiber. These are important nutrients, which your body uses during the detoxification and acid neutralization process.

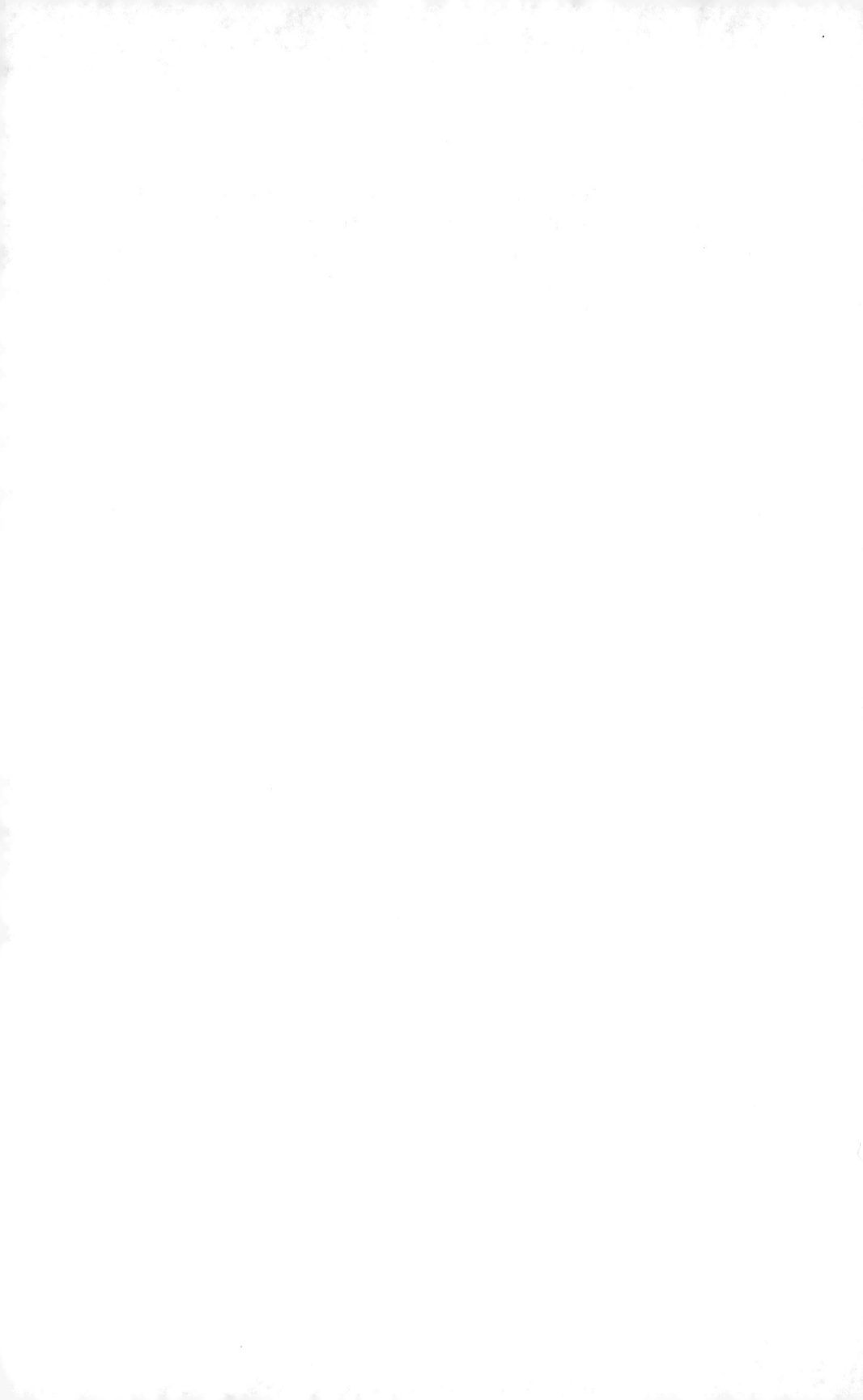

Chapter 6: Fruit Juices to Drink That Eliminate Acid

Drinking fruit juices helps to bring vitamins and minerals quickly into your blood where they can go into your body cells to give you health. Minerals quickly neutralize body acids and change your body into an alkaline state.

Juices have antibacterial action and contain digestive enzymes that help you to digest protein and fat.

Because of the vitamins, minerals, digestive enzymes, pure water, and nutrients that juices have, they have the power to cleanse your body of toxic wastes and bring you into better health.

Citrus Juices

Citrus juices are an excellent way to stimulate your colon and other parts of your body. Since your colon is less active at night, drinking juices as soon as you awaken and get up can stimulate strong peristaltic action to promote a bowel movement.

Lemon Power

For example, you would think that eating fresh lemons would be creating an acid condition in your body. But it really is the opposite. Lemons contain citric acid, but when your body uses this acid, the result is a residue that binds with acid to move your overall body into a more alkaline level.

Fruits have the power to bring your body back into the normal range of health. Many of the activities you do during the day create body acids and fruits can balance out these acids. If you do not neutralize these acids, they build up in your body and attract and create disease. The number of diseases that result from acid build in your body encompasses practically all diseases.

Mineral Binding

The only way to reduce the detrimental effects of these acids on your body is to mix them with an alkaline liquid. This is where fruits and vegetables come in. They have the power to provide what is known as "mineral binding" or "acid binding," which helps to neutralize the effect of excess body acids or excess alkaline compounds.

Fresh Lemon Juice

Fresh lemon juice is the king of fruit juices. It contains citric acid, which acts in your body in a way no other juice does. First it acts on the liver to build up its enzymes, so it can detoxify toxins in the blood. Then, it combines with calcium to form soluble chemical substances. This makes it effective in removing kidney and pancreatic stones, plaque build up along artery walls, and other calcium deposits that occur in your body.

When the liver, gallbladder, and pancreas are not working like they should, food digestion is affected. This in turn will contribute to a variety of illnesses.

Use lemons moderately since they break up oils during digestion and in our body make oils less available to your cells and joints. If you have lemon allergies or ulcers then you should avoid lemon juice.

Here's what to do:

Squeeze one lemon into a glass of warm distilled water. Drink it first thing when you wake up. Don't drink anything else for at least 1/2 hour. Let this juice get digested.

You can use a citrus press to juice the lemon or just squeeze it to get the juice out.

Organic Juices

Organic fresh made juices have cleansing and laxative action. These juices contain loads of mineral, bioflavonoids, vitamins, enzymes, antioxidants, and other nutrients. Citric fruits have citric acid and the more tart they are the more acid they have.

Fresh juice is a fast way to get all types of nutrients into the blood quickly. As juice nutrients get into your blood, they suck out toxics and build up tissue. In your colon, they destroy bacteria, feed wall tissue, pull out toxins, and activate peristaltic action.

Here are some juices to drink.

Apple juice

Drink at least 2 glasses of this juice every day. Apple juice has a high level of minerals and vitamins, which makes it ideal for neutralizing acid in your body.

Apples Juice

Because apples have a high mineral content, they are especially good for your skin, hair and fingernails. Apples that are good for juices are Granny Smith, Braeburn, Edgemont Russet, Gala, and Discovery. If apples are firm and crisp they provide good juice.

When buying apple juice, buy juice that is cloudy and not clear. This cloudy juice has more fiber and nutrients and contains a good amount of the fiber pectin.

Apple juice serves as a good base, when mixed with other juices and especially with vegetables. Most of the vitamin A lies in the skin of the apple, so it is best to juice apples without peeling.

Apple juice is good to drink when you have a cold. Its high vitamin C content helps to minimize the effects of colds and flu's. It helps improve your immune system to fight bacterial toxicity. It's a great brain tonic, since it supplies the nutrients to keep your brain healthy and active. It provides the nutrients for you to be more active.

This is one of the fruits that can be used in many ways and you still get its nutritional value. You can eat it raw, cooked, baked, juiced, jammed, or pickled.

Apple juice can remove high fever, low vitality, anemia, arthritis, pimples, blemishes, body weakness, headaches, and impure blood. Use apple juice to restore normal heart function or as a heart tonic. Use it for those that are weak, bedridden, aged, and, of course, for general health. For diabetics don't use sweet apples.

Here is a way to do a "One-day apple and apple juice fast"

Eating 3-4 apples during the day

Drink a glass of apple juice every two hours

Don't eat anything until the next morning.

Apple cider vinegar

Take 1-2 tablespoons of apple cider vinegar with 8 oz of water every day. And, add apple cider vinegar to your salad as part of your salad dressing. Just adding it to your salad will help to kill any bacteria or parasites that are in your vegetables. Apple cider vinegar will also kill any bacteria or parasite in your stomach that can cause you to have diarrhea.

Apple and Pear Juice

Prepare equal amounts of fresh apple and pear juice. Drink this combination when you first wake up and one hour before bedtime.

Juice the pears that are slightly hard. If the pear is ripe, it is best to blend it whole with apple juice to create a thick drink. Using the whole pear will give you additional fiber. Just remove the seeds but do not peel the organic type.

Pears have minerals, vitamins, and chemicals that help to clean out your colon, kidney and to regenerate your blood cells.

Apple Juice and Prune Juice

If you have a juicer you can make fresh apple juice and drink

2 - 3 glasses a day. You can also drink store-bought apple juice but try to get fresh squeezed and not the type that has been flash pasteurized or pasteurized. If you can't find fresh apple juice then use flash pasteurized.

Apple Juice, Figs and Raisins

Here's another recipe using apple juice. Use it the first thing in the morning before breakfast.

In a blender, put a cup of fresh apple juice. Add equal amounts of dry or fresh figs and raisins. Choose how many figs and raisins to use. You will need to experiment a little.

Get a consistency that is not too thick. Add a little more apple juice if needed.

Oat Milk with Fig Juice or Prune Juice

Buy oat milk at the health food store. In the morning, warm 8 oz. of oat milk and add the following:

3 oz. of fig or prune juice

Two droppers full of licorice extract.

Or you can mix one glass of 50% fig juice and 50% prune juice. Drink this first thing in the morning.

Aloe Vera Juice

This juice is use for soothing the bowel area, when it is irritated. If you have hemorrhoids it can provide you some relief. Here's how to use it. There are some aloe Vera juice drinks that you can buy at a health food store. Try them out and see what your results are. If you have aloe jell then mixt 1-2 tablespoons with 7up, some other carbonated drink, or juice. Try different aloe portions until you find one that is palatable.

Aloe Vera juice is also good if you have an ulcer or some internal lining scratch or tear. Aloe promotes the repair and regrowth of cells.

Stewed Figs

Take 10 – 12 calimyma figs and stew them in two glasses of water (16 oz) for 10 minutes. Let them sit in this water overnight.

In the morning remove the figs, warm and drink the juice. Eat the figs though out the day.

Or, prepare a blended drink of three or more figs, fresh or sun dried, and one banana

1 tablespoon of honey

one cup of rice dream

Drink first thing in the morning or any time after lunch or dinner.

Mulberry Juice

Mulberry juice has many health benefits. It is good for digestive tract illnesses. It can stimulate digestion and assimilation of nutrients in the small intestine. It is useful for older people for reliving constipation.

Mulberry contains many minerals and vitamins.

Grapefruit Juice

Instead of drinking lemon juice, drink a glass of fresh squeezed grapefruit first thing in the morning. Again, wait at least 1/2 hour before you eat anything.

If you are taking any anticonvulsant drugs, birth control pills, estrogen, protease inhibitors and even other types of drugs, avoid drinking grapefruit juice. It slows the breakdown of certain drugs, allowing them to increase in the blood to dangerous levels.

Grape fruit and Orange Juice

One excellent morning drink is a combination of grapefruit and orange juice. Just prepare a half and half drink of these citrus fruits and drink it first thing in the morning.

Pineapple Juice

Pineapple juice is another excellent juice to use frequently. It's high in potassium, which helps to strengthen the valve between the esophagus and stomach and helps to keep your nerve transmission active.

Pineapple health value comes from the enzyme bromelain that it contains. Bromelain helps keep body fluids balanced and neutral; moves an acid body to neutral and an alkaline one to neutral. It stimulates the pancreas to release its hormones. And, it has been found useful for coughs and sore throats. For some people pineapple juice affects the throat making it feel scratchy.

Grape Juice

You can add grape juice to other juices like apple to give it a different flavor. When juicing apples, you can juice a few handfuls of grapes to mix them together. Grapes have a high content of natural sugar and can give you a quick energy lift. They contain a high level of minerals and have B vitamins. You may want to grape drink from bottles, since it has a short season and in a bottle you can drink it any time. Use the darker grape drinks, because of their high anti-oxidants.

Grapes help to regulate and increase your metabolism. A low metabolism will cause you to gain weight and a high metabolism will help you burn food quicker. Because of its mineral content, it helps to build your blood and to stimulate your liver to increase its cleansing abilities. The color of fruit juices often tells you what part of the body it is good for. Red grape juice helps build your blood.

Papayas

Papaya juice is a highly curative fruit and its juice gives a powerful punch for health. It keeps arteries soft and flexible, preventing cholesterol deposits. Its digestive enzyme, pepsin, destroys the outer layer of germs, including the TB bacteria. It reduces the risk of high blood pressure, heart attacks, and improves the circulation of blood, improves liver function, restores peristaltic intestinal action, and improves vision. It is good for the aged, since it will improve their digestion allowing more nutrients to get into their body. It is a powerful meat digestive enzyme.

It is useful for skin problems and its raw milk can be applied as a face mask for blemishes, acne, leucoderma, eczema, and other face diseases. Its application can make your skin smooth and clear.

Use papaya enzymes or fresh papaya for increasing your digestive power. Papaya helps you to digest more protein, which helps you improve your cell regeneration abilities.

Citrus Fruits

Most people see citrus fruits - grapefruits, oranges, lemons, and limes – as acid food. The secret of citrus is that even though they enter your mouth as an acid food they work in your body as an alkaline residue. This residue works to eliminate acid which makes you less susceptible to disease.

The following four citruses belong to the Rutaceae family.

Grapefruit and Atherosclerosis

Grapefruit appeared around 300 years ago and no one knows how it came about. It was known as the forbidden fruit of the Caribbean.

Nutritionally, grapefruit is high in vitamin C and contains flavonoids different from the other citrus fruits. It is the flavonoid naringin that gives it its bitter taste. On its skin, the grapefruit has a phytochemical called monoterpenes, which has been found to protect against cancer. Very few people eat the skin, since it is quite bitter. However these skin phytochemicals lower blood cholesterol and clean out arterial plaque. This could be a natural remedy to reverse atherosclerosis.

Most people just eat the meat of the grapefruit, but the rind has been found, in Japan, to be high in vitamins and in nutrients that fight cancer. The rind is also bitter but you always get a little, when you peel the grapefruit.

The skin of the grapefruit can be cut into bite size pieces and dried on your counter. After a week or two, you can store them in a glass jar and chew on them, when you have an upset stomach.

Lemons and Antioxidants

Lemons go way back to 800 B.C. In the middle ages, lemons moved from the Mediterranean to Asia then to northern Africa.

Later, the Spaniards brought lemons to South American.

Lemons were used to treat and cure scurvy in the 16th Century and in Roman times people used them as a poison antidote. Lemons also have monoterpenes like grapefruit. These monoterpenes are powerful antioxidants and in combination with vitamin C have cancer prevention and fighting abilities.

Lemons are considered acidic but when their nutrients enter the body and are used up, the residue becomes alkaline. This residue becomes available to neutralize body acids. Most people have acid bodies and lack minerals to adjust their bodies back to normal or alkaline. So, lemons and other citric fruits should be eaten daily, even if you have arthritis.

Limes and Monoterpenes

Limes have similar properties as lemons, since they too contain monoterpenes. English sailors, to prevent scurvy, also used them. You can eat the other skin to get the most health benefit from limes. Throw them in a blender with other juices to get a strong citrus drink.

Oranges and D-limonene

Oranges existed in China in 2400 B.C. Through trading, oranges were spread throughout Europe and the rest of the world. Oranges are high in vitamin C and their skin contains a good amount of monoterpenes and oil called d-limonene.

Use citrus fruits daily for their vitamin C, phytonutrients, and antioxidants that protect you from cancer and other diseases. Use them for arthritis to neutralize and remove acids that surround joints and cause inflammation.

Chapter 7: Special Nutrient That Give Powerful Health

Here is a list of special drinks and nutrients that will give you powerful health. Look over this list and implement some of them and try out others to see which ones give you the best results.

Grapefruit Whole Leaf Aloe Vera Juice

Combine 6 oz. grapefruit and add 2 oz. of aloe Vera and then add more aloe or less as you get use to the taste.

Another way to use this combination is to use aloe Vera capsules and drink them with 6 – 8 oz. of grapefruit juice.

Aloe Vera has anti-inflammatory properties and can heal open wounds by promoting cell regeneration. Grapefruit contain vitamin C and plenty of bioflavonoids that can prevent tissue damage from free radicals.

Honey

It has been found by the United States Department of Agriculture nutritionist Richard J. Wood that the glucose in honey can increase your absorption of calcium by up to 25%. It can also increase the absorption of zinc and magnesium.

Using honey for asthma and other respiratory illness makes sense, since honey has an antibacterial effect. Honey draws out the moisture from bacteria and kills them dead.

Use honey that is unfiltered, unheated, and dark. This type of honey contains more levulose, a type of sugar molecule that is absorbed into the blood slowly and does not cause the blood sugar to rise too fast.

Here is a recipe that has been used by many people and that you can use when you have to deal with asthma every day. It reduces inflammation and continual coughing.

Cut up 3-5 slices of onions

Cut up a clove of garlic

Place this in 16 oz. of Irish moss jelly and simmer for 30 minutes. After it cools add 4 – 5 ounces of local organic raw honey. Mix in well and,

Take one teaspoon every other hour and one teaspoon of pure honey every alternative hour.

Another way of using honey, garlic and onions is to soak slices of onions and garlic in honey overnight. The next day, stir the mixture to spread the onion and garlic juices into the honey.

Or, if you have a juicer or a garlic press you can press out the onion and garlic juice and let this sit overnight in some honey.

The next day, take this mixture 3 – 4 times during day.

Using eucalyptus honey makes this remedy even more powerful since eucalyptus leaves have healing effects for asthma and helps to break down mucus that forms in the bronchioles.

Foods High in Magnesium

Chlorophyll is high in magnesium and chlorophyll comes in capsules and liquid. Drink 2 oz. or less of chlorophyll liquid daily by combining it with the juice of one lemon and 6-8 oz. of distilled water. Do this first thing in the morning.

MSM

MSM stands for methyl sulfonyl methane. MSM is organic sulfur. It provides many benefits in the body and is widely used as an anti-inflammatory and is especially useful for arthritis pain. MSM is used in all body cells and tissue including joint tissue. As a needed body nutrient, take 2000 mg per day using MSM torpedoes.

Antioxidants

The body produces antioxidants to neutralize free radicals that become excessive in your body. Free radicals have a damaging effect on the tissue they encounter as they float throughout your body. Left uncheck they cause numerous deadly diseases.

The way the body takes care of this threat is to create antioxidants. However the body's antioxidants are not always enough to capture all these free radicals. This is because free radical can be created in numerous ways and can be found in food, air, water, and personal products.

Free radicals are also created with emotional states, such as anger, fear, depression, jealousy, and anxiety.

The result is that your body needs help to neutralize these free radicals, and this is where fruits, vegetables, special nutrients, vitamins, and minerals come in. Produce is packed with antioxidants. Using them to neutralize free radicals has become a necessity.

There are many minerals and vitamins that are classified as antioxidants. These are vitamins A, C, E, and selenium. Other antioxidants are bioflavonoids, carotenoids, isoflavones, all minerals, allium vegetables like garlic and onions, bilberry, coenzyme Q10, cruciferous vegetables, Ginkgo Biloba, glutathione, lipoic acid, superoxide dismutase, and melatonin.

Antioxidants and Phytonutrients

Phytochemicals or phytonutrients are mostly found in the skin of fruits and are considered antioxidants. These nutrients give the fruit its color. Fruits also contain fundamental antioxidants, like vitamin A, C, E, beta carotene, zinc and selenium. Try to buy organic fruits so you can eat the skins without worry. In some fruits there are more nutrients on the skin than in the fruit.

Other antioxidants that you may have heard of are carotenoids, lutein, lycopene, sod, and glutathione, anthocyanins, and lipoic acid. The list is in the hundreds.

The discovery of antioxidants and their importance in preventing disease is one of the century's most important health discoveries. For this reason eating fruits and vegetables is probably the most important thing you can do to prevent disease and improve your health.

As a start, fruits and vegetables should consist of 40% to 50% of the food you eat. For most people, it is around 20%.

Just work at it little by little and eat more produce as the weeks pass.

Phytonutrients are special nutrients that are found in fruits and other plants. In plants they protect them from disease, insects, excess heat, UV rays, poisons, pollutants, injury and drought.

Phytonutrients have been found to be beneficial to human life. They contain chemicals that are useful in treating and preventing diseases such as cancer, diabetes, cardiovascular disease, and hypertension.

The phytonutrients consists of many groups, but the most important groups are the phytosterols and phytohormones. These sterols are precursors to your human sterols.

Bioflavonoids

Bioflavonoids are also antioxidants that are chemicals, which come from water soluble colors found in fruits, vegetables, grains, leaves, and barks. Because they are found in a variety of plant food, they come in different chemical forms and concentrations.

Some of the bioflavonoids are more powerful in destroying free radicals then the standbys, vitamin C and E. Some well known flavonoids are catechins, reserveratrol, and proanthocyanidines.

Chinese acid reflux remedies

Here is a Chinese remedy that helps to strengthen and tone up the stomach lining. Using this remedy will help you to normalize your stomach function.

This remedy is discussed in Richard Lucas's book, Secrets of the Chinese Herbalist, 1977.

"Step 1: Put one-half cup of white rice in a flat bowl. Pour in enough water to barely cover the rice. Let stand overnight so that the rice can completely absorb the water. In the morning if there is any water still standing in the bowl, drain it off. Put the rice in a dry frying pan, and gradually heat it until the pan is quite hot. Use a spatula, and keep turning the rice slowly so it doesn't burn. When the rice is parched dry and golden brown, put it in a glass jar and cap tightly against moisture.

Step 2: Bring one cup of water to a boil; add one teaspoon of the parched rice and a small piece of ginger root. Boil for one minute, and then turn off the burner and let stand for five minutes. Then strain and take one teacupful once or twice a day."

Po Chai

Po Chai is another Chinese natural remedy. It is a tiny pill and can be purchased in any Chinese herbal shop. It's designed to give you relief for acid reflux and gas bloating. Use warm water or tea to drink it down. It works in about 15 minutes and can be taken every two hours, if necessary.

Bye-Lori II™

Bye-Lori is special formulation to help cure stomach problems such as ulcers, heartburn, and more. It can restore stomach function back to normal. It is designed to kill the helicobacter pylori bacteria that causes ulcers, destroys good bacteria and upset stomach function.

Kyolic

Kyolic is aged, powder garlic. It has an antibacterial quality and is used to kill bad bacterial, Candida, and helibactor pylori, which can be a source for acid reflux.

Probiotics

Use friendly bacteria like L. acidophilus in capsules 2 – 4 times a day between meals.

Ginger Root

Drink one cup of ginger root daily. Buy it fresh and grate one teaspoon and place it into one cup of boiling distilled water. Then steep it for 10 minutes. You can add a little honey if it is too strong for you.

Dandelion Root

Drink one cup of dandelion root every day. You can buy the root at a health food store that sells herbs. You can get dandelion root at various health stores that sell loose herbs. Try creating a tea of ginger root and dandelion root with honey.

Sweet potatoes

Sweet potatoes can help get you regular. Prepare sweet potatoes just before you go to bed. Boil or bake the sweet potatoes. Then, eat them with some milk, salt, or honey. This mixture for sure will get your bowels moving.

16. Mace, Nutmeg, and Slippery Elm

Here is a natural remedy that uses mace and nutmeg, which has a history of treating indigestion, acid stomach, heartburn, acid reflux, stomach gas, and vomiting.

Here's how to use it with half and half and slippery elm root herb. Slippery elm herb can be purchase in any herb store in powder.

1 teaspoon of slippery elm bark

a pinch of nutmeg

a pinch of mace

add distilled water to make a smooth slurry

heat a pint of half and half to boil

pull half and half from stove and add herb slurry

stir in herb slurry

Allow this mixture to cool. Drink up to ½ cup at a time. Store the unused portion in the refrigerator. When drinking the next cup, warm this mixture up.

Acid reflux and heartburn require alkaline nutrients to provide relief. These 4 natural remedies, when prepared properly, will give you the relief you need from these conditions. Try them and you will be surprised how well they work.

No need to use antacids, which have unwanted side effects and contain aluminum. It has been associated with senility and Alzheimer's disease.

Anise and peppermint

Here's a tea that you can make to help you with acid reflux or heartburn. It will help you reduce the amount of acid you have in your stomach. Mix together equal amounts of aniseed, peppermint and lavender. Make an infusion of this tea:

boil 2 ½ cup distilled water

pour this water over a heaping teaspoon of the herbal mixture

let this tea sit for 3- 5 minutes

strain the tea and add a little bit of honey, if you like. Place this tea into a thermos

Drink up to 8 oz. in the morning and 8 oz. in the evening to get relief of acid reflux.

Aniseed or anise – is a powerful herb that helps in digestive conditions and has many other benefits for your body. Use only the ash-colored anise called green anise, European anise or sweet anise. There are two other types of anise, star anise and caraway, which should not be used here.

Peppermint – is another powerful herb for stomach conditions or heartburn. It helps in digestion, stomach distension, cramps, ulcers, and gas.

Betaine, Pepsin, and Papaya digestive enzymes

As you get older, your stomach weakens in its ability to produce hydrochloric acid to digest protein. It is undigested protein that leads to acid reflux or heartburn. Use digestive enzymes that contain Betaine, pepsin, or HCl with each meal to make sure you digest all of your protein.

Papaya digestive enzymes, which contain papain, are also excellent for protein digestion and you can use them with each meal. Use 500mg or more of papaya enzymes per meal.

Vitamin B12 Deficiency Triggers Anemia

When the level of Vitamin B12 is reduced to below what is needed in the body, a vitamin deficiency results and triggers iron Deficiency Anemia. Vitamin B12 is used to make red blood cells in the bone marrow. B12 injections may be necessary in case B12 capsules have no significant effect.

Iron Deficiency Anemia is due to the insufficient intake, or absorption of Iron. It includes the failure to replace losses from menstruation or from diseases. Since Iron is an essential element in hemoglobin, its low levels will result in a weakened incorporation of hemoglobin in red blood cells.

In pre-menopausal women, blood is lost during their menstrual periods. Accordingly, the resulting Iron deficiency, especially in teenage girls, causes poor performance in school.

On a worldwide scale, Iron deficiency is the most prevalent deficiency state.

Zinc

Zinc is useful for cell production. It helps create new cells and is needed for healing, growth, or pregnancy.

When one is wounded or cut, zinc helps replicate cells quickly by creating collagen to heal the wound fast.

During their menstrual period, women can be irritable and give off the stay-away-from-me reaction. Zinc helps them normalize their mood.

Second only to calcium, Zinc is the most deficient mineral in a woman's diet. Thus, women need to use a supplement of at least 15 to 30 mg. of zinc every day.

Manganese

Manganese is called the "love element" because people who lack it show signs of meanness, vindictiveness, lacking love, and are anti-social. It is found in the linings of the brain, in the nerves, in the lining of the heart, and in the blood. It helps carry oxygen from the lungs to the cells.

Manganese strengthens the lining of the bronchioles and makes them more elastic.

Manganese works with certain enzymes to help cells use fat, protein and carbohydrate. It helps protect the cells from free radical damage.

There are indications that people with asthma are low in manganese. Your diet should include those foods that are high in manganese.

Peas, beans, blueberries, Missouri black walnuts, almonds, pecans sesame seeds, buckwheat, cardamom, marjoram, rye bread, pumpernickel bread, and steel cut oats, apples, apricots, black-eyed peas, celery, parsley, watercress, wheat bran, wheat germ, whole grains, avocados, and cantaloupes.

Pineapple is another source high in manganese. It also is high in vitamins A and C.

Taking electrolyte manganese liquid will also supply you with ionic manganese that is ready to use by your body.

MSM, MethylSulfonylMethane

MSM is organic sulphur. It is now widely available in capsule, pill, or powder form and in different purity grades.

In their book, MSM The Definitive Guide, 2003, Stanley W. Jacob, M.D., FL.A.C.S. and Jeremy Appleton, N. D., talk about an individual that came to their clinic with asthma,

"AA had been hospitalized for seven months (multiple admissions) for asthma. She experienced frequent attacks, beginning with wheezing, coughing, and shortness of breath: this was followed by respiratory distress. Her therapy had included antihistaminic agents, theophylline, and corticosteroids.

We administered oral MSM, starting with ¼ teaspoon of powder (approximately 1 gram) twice daily. We gradually increased her dosage to 8 grams per day. She remains on this dosage at the time of this writing and has not required hospitalization for three years."

MSM is an anti-inflammatory and is used to reduce arthritic pain. But it is useful in reducing inflammation in any part of the body including inflammation of the bronchioles.

MSM helps the body keep its acid-alkaline balance. It also

helps in the creation and regeneration of the body's tissues. MSM is found in every body cell and helps keep cells soft, so nutrients can easily go into the cell and waste can easily come out. This easy movement of chemicals, in and out of the cell, helps the body recover from illness quicker and helps make your body healthier.

Here's how to use MSM:

During the first week: Take 3 grams or 1 gram with each meal

During the second week: Take 4 – 6 grams or 2 grams per meal.

You can take more MSM and you can reduce the amount of MSM you take when you start having to many bowel movements.

Mullein Tea

Mullein tea has been found to be useful in asthma, if taken every day. It is slow to show results, but continual use will provide lasting results in asthma relief.

Make a tea out of dried or fresh leaves. Simmer for 10 – 15 minutes for a strong tea.

Oxygen

When you have an asthma attack, your body is struggling for oxygen. Here are some things that you can add to your diet that can bring in more oxygen into your body cells.

Vitamin E – use 400 IU

Fish oil – take as directed on the bottle
Digestive enzymes with HCl – use 1-2 capsules per meal
Relaxation

People have lessened their asthma attacks by learning self-hypnosis and relaxation. By learning yoga breathing exercises you can improve your asthma and have less attacks.

In the book, High Speed Healing, 1991, by Prevention Editors, they report that Dr. Schenkel says,

"Short of medication, what I often recommend for asthma is relaxation. What happens with asthma is you're hungry for air so you panic and the panic tends to make asthma worse. Simply relaxing the way you usually relax is one of the best treatments you can give yourself – and relaxation can help soothe an asthma attack in about 15 to 20 minutes."

Dr. Bach has developed a blend of flower remedies that helps you relax when you have anxiety as when you feel an asthma attack coming. He has developed an array of flower remedies that help with emotional and psychological problems.

The flower remedies to use for asthma are found under the names:

Calming Essence,

Rescue Remedy

Five-Flower Formula

Emergency Stress Relief Formula

Here's how to use them. Place 4 drops under the tongue and

hold there for a minute, so that the flower nutrients are absorbed into the blood. You can also add four drops into a glass of distilled water and sip it slowly.

The intent of using these flower remedies is to calm you, when you feel anxious or to calm you when you feel an asthma attack looming.

Ruby Reds

Ruby Reds is a special powder that contains all of the vitamins and minerals you need to keep healthy. It contains powders of many fruits and vegetables which provide fiber, probiotics, and digestive enzymes. You will enhance your blood cleansing by using Ruby Reds powder, since it has the nutrients you need in your cells and in your lymph liquids to neutralize waste and acids. You can get all this from the juices you drink, but Ruby Reds gives you additional nutrients to cleanse out your body.

The way to use Ruby Reds is to add one capful of the powder into the juice that you will be drinking for the day. Or, if you make a smoothie, just add one capful to it. Ruby Reds has natural sugar so the taste of your drink with Ruby Reds will be enjoyable.

Chlorophyll

Use chlorophyll as a liquid. Chlorophyll is the blood source of plants. It is very similar in chemical structure to our blood. It will elevate your blood count and will work to neutralize and detoxify your body toxins. Using chlorophyll will reduce your body odor and stool smell. It gets into your blood and is used by all of your cells.

Cayenne

Cayenne is effective in producing peristalsis in your colon by aiding in digestion and stimulating elimination. It can be used regularly and when needed for constipation. Cayenne pepper is known to help thin the blood. So, it is good for improving the blood circulation.

Cayenne is available in capsules of different strengths, from 5,000 heat units (HU) to 100,000 and even higher. In addition, cayenne when used with other herbs helps to deliver these herbs more efficiently to where they are needed in your body.

Start with one capsule of 40,000 HU and always take it after you eat. You will feel a hot or slight burning feeling in the upper stomach and that's when you know it's working. The feeling is like when you get heartburn. This burning sensation will pass as your body gets use to you using cayenne.

Do not use cayenne seeds, as they can be toxic. If you are pregnant or breast-feeding do not take cayenne supplements. Use cayenne only as showed on containers and only as capsules.

Cayenne has the ability to block the ulcer producing effect of NSAIDS. It also has shown to increase the body's absorption of theopylline, a drug used to treat asthma.

In his book, Left for Dead, Dick Quinn tells how Cayenne pepper saved his life after coronary bypass surgery failed to restore his health. In this book, Shannon Quinn, say, "One of the most effective stimulants, mostly, cayenne targets the digestive and the circulatory system. Cayenne regulates blood pressure, strengthens the pulse, feeds the heart, lowers cholesterol, and thins the blood. It cleanses the circulatory system, heals ulcers, stops hemorrhaging, speeds healing of wounds, rebuilds damaged tissue, eases congestion, aids digestion, regulates elimination, relieves arthritis and rheumatism, prevents the spread of infection and numbs pain."

Use the recommended dose shown on the bottle of cayenne you use.

You can also add cayenne pepper into other foods. Add cayenne to soups, salads, and other food you like.

In soups or salads break open a cayenne capsule and mix it in. You can add 1 – 2 capsules but first start with 1/4 or 1/2 capsule so you can get use to the hot taste. Even with ¼ capsule, a soup will be hot.

If you are pregnant, it is considered safe to use cayenne.

Enzymes for children

Digestive enzymes can be given to infants, toddlers, and young children. All tests show that there are no side effects when children take digestive enzymes. Digestive enzymes can be mixed with food, water, or juice.

There is no addiction to using enzymes. Once you stop using them, your body just takes over and continues to produce them. Using enzymes saves your own power to create them later in life.

Using enzymes

It's best to use plant enzyme supplements. These enzymes are more stable over a wider pH and temperature range. They function very well in the high acidic pH of your stomach. Animal or pancreatic enzymes do not function in the stomach. These types of enzymes need to be coated so they pass the stomach and reach the small intestines where they work well in a high alkaline pH.

Remember there are two types of enzymes that you can purchase – digestive and systemic. You can use digestive enzymes with the food you eat and take the systemic enzymes between meals.

Take 2 – 4 digestive enzymes around 15 minutes before you meal. For small meals use 1–2 capsules. For meals where you eat fruits and vegetable, again only take 1-2 capsules. If you forget to take them before your meal take them with your meal or after. Also take 2 capsules between meals to help build up your body stores of enzymes.

By supplying your body with external digestive enzymes, it allows your body to concentrate its energy in creating enzymes for use in other parts of your body. Taking enzymes between meals on an empty stomach helps to strengthen your immune system and to neutralize free radicals, toxins, and undigested protein that gets into your blood.

Digestive enzymes

Your blood needs good nutrition and it gets it when you properly digest your food and absorb it through your small and large intestine. By the time you are 30 years, your digestive abilities decreases considerably. To improve your digestion, you need to take digestive enzymes at the start or after each meal.

Use a broadband digestive enzyme that contains amylase, protease, and lipase. If you are over 60, start testing to see if you need Betaine HCL. The amount and strength of your stomach acid, HCL, decreases as you age and your ability to digest proteins and fats decreases. Without a good amount of HCL which has a pH of 1.5-3, you cannot properly process protein and process calcium, B12, and iron. Even more important is that the lack of HCL limits the destruction of bad bacteria and micro-organisms you eat - Salmonella, E. coli , and C. difficile .

Chamomile tea

When you have reflux symptoms, first use chamomile tea. This tea soothes the stomach.

Peppermint tea

There is some controversy about using peppermint tea for acid reflux, but many people use it to settle their stomach. By all means buy peppermint tea bags and try them out. But, there are other herbs to use that are just as effective for acid reflux

Cinnamon and Cardamom tea

Make a tea of cinnamon or of cardamom to help alleviate heartburn.

Cinnamon

Cinnamon has many medicinal uses aside from being great for various pastries. It has an antiseptic effect and has been historically used for colds and flu's. It has fighting power against Candida albicans and has the ability to settle acidic stomachs.

Here's how to use cinnamon for an acid stomach or heartburn:

Toast raisin bread

Butter the raisin bread

Sprinkle cinnamon on the bread

Sprinkle cardamon on the bread

When you eat this toasted bread, chew slowly and completely before swallowing to allow the digestive juices in your mouth to start breaking down this food.

Cardamon, which is found in India, has been used successful in treating Celiac disease, which is intolerance to gluten found in most bread.

Echinacea

Echinacea helps to elevate your immune system. It has many actions in your body that will help to eliminate illness and infections. It is a natural antibiotic, and has anti-viral and anti-inflammatory action, so it will help to stop your ear aches, slow down cold or flu conditions, and help illnesses of various kinds.

Since your immune system is involved in fighting and removing pathogens and toxics, the less work it has to do the stronger it will be. Echinacea and many other herbs and nutrients can help you eliminate some of the conditions that weaken your immune system.

Here are some important activities that Echinacea performs to strengthen your immune system:

Stimulates phagocytosis T-cell formation, which fight pathogen

Increases the ability of white blood cells to surround and destroy bacterial and viral pathogens.

cleanses the blood

Works like penicillin in the body with no side effects

treats strep throat and lymph gland infections

expels poisons and toxins

Cleans out the stomach of toxic matter

Use Echinacea in connection with other medication or natural remedies that you are using. The actual doses are defined on the bottle it comes in. For adults 50 drops in water should be taken 4 to 5 times a day. For children use 1/3 this amount.

Melatonin

So, what does melatonin have to do with hair loss? In clinical studies with rats, melatonin was shown to extent their life expectancy by 15 to 30%. Those rats that took melatonin had better fur for a long period of time than those rats that did not take melatonin. It is the pineal gland, in the brain, that secretes melatonin. This secretion slowly decreases as your body ages. It appears that when the pineal gland slows its melatonin output, it is telling the body to age. And, as you age and various body systems and organs deteriorate, you start to lose more hair.

You can keep your hair for a longer time in your life when you take melatonin. But, not by just taking melatonin, you must take other supplements and eat the food that keeps your whole body healthy and strong.

A typical melatonin dose most people take is 1-5 mg. Some people have experience headaches when they take melatonin. Since melatonin is a hormone, it may upset the balance your hormones. If you get headaches, just don't use it or decrease the dose.

Perhaps one reason melatonin works so good is that it works in conjunction with the thymus gland, the master immunity gland, to help protect you from illness and disease.

Fiber - Fiber is critical to your health. Many people don't eat fruits and/or vegetables. This is a big mistake because this is the only way you can get naturally balanced vitamins, minerals and nutrients that your body needs. Yes you can take supplements, but this is not the best way to get your nutrients.

Lack of fiber affects digestion and assimilation of nutrients. It also is necessary for eliminating toxins and excess nutrients that your body does not need. When you don't eat enough fiber, food stays longer in your intestinal tract causing toxins and bacteria to form. These toxins can be absorbed into your blood affecting the quality of your blood and function of your cells.

Lack of fiber in your diet affects hair growth, because the quality of nutrients in your blood decreases.

You main source of fiber should be from the following produce. You can get fiber from grains, but cooked they have no enzymes.

- Raw wheat germ
- brewer's yeast or nutritional yeast
- lecithin
- carrot juice
- vegetable oils
- honey
- kelp
- sunflower seeds or meal
- nuts
- all sorts of raw fruits that are grown in your location
- all sorts of raw vegetables that are grown in your location

Probiotics

Probiotics refers to live good bacteria that you have in your stomach, intestines, and colon. It is live bacteria that you can supplement your diet with. You have over 500 species of good and bad bacteria spread throughout your gastrointestinal tract, starting in your mouth and ending in your anus. These bacteria are at constant war with each other, each trying to dominate. The most important thing about bacteria is that you must have more good bacteria than bad, so that the good bacteria can maintain control of your gastrointestinal tract and provide you with good health.

If you have history of using antibiotics or have recently used them, then you need to use a good probiotics for a least a month. Using antibiotics kills both good and bad bacteria, allowing bad bacteria to take over your gastrointestinal tract and thereby producing toxins and excretions that are bad for your blood and body functions.

Once bad bacteria takes over it is hard to re-establish your good bacteria, but using a good probiotics can help you do this. Using probiotics helps your digestion and makes your intestinal tract more alkaline, making it difficult for bad bacteria to thrive.

Good bacterial also helps you create vitamin K, B12, and Biotin.

Here is a list of good bacteria that you can find in supplements, where the L stands for Lactobacillus.

L. Acidophilus

L. Bifidus

L. Bulgaricus

S. Thermophilus

L. Casei

The most common good bacteria are the first three in this list. When you buy probiotics only buy a supplement with a few strains of good bacteria, since the compete with each other to take over the intestinal area.

CHAPTER 8: SUPPLEMENTS YOU NEED MORE OF

Vitamins do not provide energy for the body, they are not found in our tissue, and they do not build cells, but help in converting the food we eat over to nutrients that our body can use. This means they help enzymes break down our food - protein, fat, and carbohydrates. Your body can make only a few vitamins.

The Next Best Mineral Supplements

If electrolytic minerals, in liquid form, are not available, use chelated minerals. These minerals are attached to amino acids making them magnetic, which allow them to flow right through your intestinal walls without having to be digested. Look for minerals such as,

- Calcium aspertate
- Calcium gluconate
- Calcium Citrate
- Zinc aspartate

Quercetin

Quercetin is a flavonoid. A flavonoid is the chemical in fruits and flowers that gives them their color. Quercetin has a high activity against asthma and acts somewhat similar to the drug Cromolyn. What quercetin does is block the release of histamine from "mast cells." When it does this, it substantially reduces the irritation and inflammation reaction to allergens.

Also, quercetin blocks another inflammatory substance that is release by the "mast cells" called leukotriene. This substance is a thousand times more powerful and harmful than histamine.

Since the body does not readily absorb quercetin, it is best to take it with bromelain to improve its absorption. You can look on the internet for the Quercetin Bromelain combination.

Quercetin twice a day at 300mg

Vitamin A

Vitamin A should never be taken by itself. It should be used with other vitamins or taken with food or with fruit snacks.

When taken alone, Vitamin A will putrefy in your colon creating toxic chemicals that may get into your blood.

Vitamin A is an important vitamin, which helps to improve your immunity. Since your colon is an important part of your immune system, it is recommended you eat those foods, which are high in Vitamin A or to use Vitamin A supplements.

Vitamin A also helps you absorb protein in your small intestine. Any protein that is not absorbed will move into your colon undigested. In this form and in your colon, this protein decays producing highly toxic material that can cause serious illness over time.

If you are pregnant or planning to get pregnant, do not take more than 5000 IU each day to avoid birth defects. If you have any liver disease, consult your doctor before taking vitamin A.

Vitamin A Emulsion

Use 50,000 IU for the first month, then drop down to 30,000 IU for two weeks and then to 20,000 IU after that.

Vitamin A and E

Vitamin A and E are used to control and stop infections from growing. You can take up to 50,000IU of vitamin A and 500 to 600 IU of vitamin E. For children use around 1/3 the dose or you can use one teaspoon of cod liver oil. Both vitamin A and E enhance the immune system.

B-Vitamins

B-vitamins are needed to feed your colon wall nerves, so they can flexible and move naturally. Without these vitamins your colon walls cannot move in a natural rhythm.

Eat less sugar and sweets since these foods use up B-vitamins when being digested.

Men need more B vitamins than women. And, there are a lot of body conditions that destroy these vitamins, such as stress or excess exercising. Eating processed foods will make you deficient in B vitamins, since B vitamins are needed in digesting processed foods.

Since B vitamins are water soluble, they are easily lost from vegetables or grains that are heated, boiled or over cooked.

Take Thiamine (B1) 100-300 mg each day since it helps to correct constipation by stimulating peristalsis.

Inositol – Helps stimulate your colon walls. Inadequate inositol is associated with constipation. Drinking too much coffee reduces inositol from the body. Use 100 – 300 mg each day.

Folic Acid - If you have leg cramps, you may need folic acid. In this case take 400-800 IU of folic acid each day.

Pantothenic acid – Taking 5 mg to 3 grams before bed, improves the health of your colon.

Vitamin B complex

The B vitamins assist immune function and are necessary for ear healing. It also helps to relieve your ear pressure. Use the 50 vitamin B complex three times a day.

Vitamin C

Taking Vitamin C will help to keep you regular. It is a gentle laxative when taken in high doses. When you become constipated, increase your use of Vitamin C. Add 500 mg each day until you reach 5000 mg. At some point, you may experience diarrhea. When this happens, just back off on the dose by 500 mg. When your constipation is cleared go back to your maintenance dose.

Using vitamin C in doses greater than 500 mg is not recommended, if you have kidney stone, liver disease, or gout.

Vitamin C may increase your absorption of aluminum, if you

are taking antacids. Take vitamin C two hours before taking antacids to prevent this problem.

Recommend vitamin C dose is 2000 – 3000 mg each day taken with meals. Pregnant women can take up to 500 mg each day.

Vitamin C is important is reducing asthma attacks. It is able to stop bronchial constriction and reduce histamine production and release. It also helps to lower histamine levels, after histamine is released into the blood. So take between 2000 mg to 4000 mg per day. Spread them out to 3 times per day with each meal. Use Ester C, if other Vitamin C supplements give you stomach problems.

Vitamin D

Vitamin D is necessary to improve your immune system, so it can fight inflammation. You can get the proper dose of Vitamin D by going out in the sun everyday for about 20 to 30 minutes.

Vitamin E

Vitamin E is good protection against heart disease and cancer. Take up to 400IU daily.

A deficiency in vitamin E is rare. However, there is a correlation between Anemia and Vitamin E deficiency. Those who are diagnosed with anemic are also found to be deficient in Vitamin E.

Vitamin E works with vitamins A and C and selenium in acting as anti-oxidants against free radicals. By reducing the effects of free radicals, this action improves the strength of your immune system.

Folic Acid

Folic acid is needed for blood cell replication, growth and regeneration. Fruits, vegetables and grains are high in folic acid. If you do not eat plenty of these daily, you may not be getting the 40mcg. of folic acid recommend by the FDA.

Severe folic deficiency is rare, but mild to borderline conditions may exist in many individuals. The elderly are at risk for folic deficiency since they,

- Eat more cooked food which loses folic acid
- Use more drugs, anticonvulsant, anticancer, cortisone, sleeping pills, or sufa drugs that interfere with folate nutrition,
- Lack the ability to absorb folate from food as they age, or can deplete their folic acid quickly.

Generally, you cannot get the amount of folic acid you need by increasing your intake of fruits and vegetables. You will need to take a folic acid supplement.

Folic acid works with 2 different enzymes to make your DNA - the material that contains your genetic code.

Folic acid also plays an important role in the development of babies. Folic acid deficiency can produce life-threatening defects in the brain and spine. This defect usually occurs during the first two weeks of pregnancy.

Another benefit of folic acid is that it helps prevent arteriosclerosis, hardening of the arteries, by changing the harmful amino acid homocysteine into a form less damaging to the arteries.

Using birth control pills can reduce folic acid in the body, as well as Vitamin B12. Doctors recommend a minimum of 40mcg. of folic acid daily.

Organic Sodium

The difference between organic sodium and inorganic sodium, table salt, is organic sodium is found in fruits and vegetables. It is alive and has electromagnetic energy and frequencies that your body uses to energizing itself. But inorganic sodium found in table salt and in many other processed foods is considered dead food. Table salt is not alive and is not the correct sodium that the body needs for good health, but your body will still use it as a substitute when you lack salt.

CHAPTER 9: BODY CYCLE YOU SHOULD KNOW ABOUT

Natural Body Cycles

Most of you are looking for ways to improve your health, lose weight, or get rid of an illness that you have. If you have acid reflux or heartburn, then you might be looking for a way to prevent it from coming back, after you have completed a colon cleanse

Here's some information that will help you achieve these results. It is call "Using the Natural Body Cycles" for achieving maximum health.

By learning how to assist your "Natural Body Cycles", you will be in tune with what your body is doing to maintain your health.

Getting in tune with your Natural Body Cycles requires change in the way you eat. Since all of us are addicted to the way we eat, it is, sometimes, difficult to change these habits. But if you are serious about what you want, this is one of the best ways to get good health.

Using this method to gain better health, you will experience side effects because you will be eliminating more body toxins and body wastes. The side effects may be headaches, stomach upsets, body pain, or similar types of symptoms. These conditions will not last and will disappear as you get rid of more toxins. So if you experience these side effects, don't let them stop you from moving forward on this eating pattern.

Here are the 3 natural body cycles:

Cycle 1 time period: 4 a.m. to 12 noon

This cycle is the time where your body is eliminating toxins, acids, wastes, and derby by urine, bowel movements, and other secretions.

Cycle 2 time period: 12 noon to 8 p.m.

This is the time when your body should be taking in food and digesting

Cycle 3 time period: 8 p.m. to 4 a.m.

This is the time your body is absorbing and using the food you have eaten during the 12 noon to 8 p.m. period.

Here's how to use cycle 1:

Breakfast

During the elimination cycle, 4 a.m. to 12 noon, eat and drink only fruits and their juices or drink vegetable juices. For breakfast eat a bowl of fruit or have a fruit smoothie made with apple juice and fruits in season.

Before noontime eat fruits as snack. Forty-five minutes before noon eat your last fruit. You can eat and drink all the fruits and juices you want up to noontime.

Bananas, oranges, apricots, strawberries, melon,

watermelons, apples, peaches, nectarines, and so on.

Eat all melons together and not with other fruit and wait 1/2 hour before eating other fruit. Melons require their specific enzymes to be digested in your stomach, so other fruit eaten with melons will just sit in your stomach waiting to be digested.
By eating in this way you are assisting your body's elimination cycle. This helps your body to eliminate toxins and acids from your body and blood. It is these toxins and acids that make you sick and overweight.

Solid Food

Eating solid food for breakfast – eggs potatoes, rice, meat, cereal, milk, and so on - interfere with your body's elimination cycle and eventually leads to sickness and excess weight. It takes over 3 hours to digest heavy and solid food. The food you should be eating, in the morning, should digest quickly to help remove toxins, acids, and waste from your body that accumulate during the night.

Heavy food slows down the elimination of toxins from your body and this causes more toxins to remain in your body. These stored toxins are converted to fat and acids. Acids are the main cause of most illnesses and so you want to have an alkaline body. Fruits and vegetables give you an alkaline body.

It takes up to 1 ½ hour or so to digest fruits and fruit juices. Because of this, they help to cleanse your body of waste, during the morning. Fruits are 70% water just like your body.

So if you are not already having fruit and fruit juices for

breakfast and snacks, start slowing changing your habits, if you want to lose weight and feel better.

Now, one other thing, don't eat fruits and juices with your lunch or dinner meals.

Natural Body Cycle 2

Cycle 2 time period: 12 noon to 8 p.m.

This is the time when your body should be taking in food and digesting it.

During this period is time to eat solid food. What you eat has to be in alignment with what your stomach can do.

Here's how your stomach works. In generally it can only digest one solid food at a time.

A solid food is one that does not contain 70% water, like fruits and vegetables do, and whose water has been eliminated by heat or other food processes, in other words cooked. Your stomach can only work on one solid food at a time, so your lunch and dinner should only have one solid food. A lunch can consist of chicken and a green salad, fish and a green salad, tuna and a green salad, shrimp and a green salad, beef and a green salad.

Mixing a protein meal with carbohydrates is giving the stomach two solid foods at the same time, which require different concentrations of digestive juices.
Giving the stomach more than it can handle interrupts the elimination cycle 1 and reduces the energy that you need for the elimination cycle.

Any eating habit that disrupts cycle 2, the eating and digestion cycle, affects the other cycles. Here's how you can help your body's cycle 2 to be more effective.

Eat only one solid food with vegetables during lunch or dinner. Lunch can be one meat or seafood with a fresh vegetable salad.

Limit the amount of water you drink during your eating. Excess water will dilute your digestive acids and slow down digestion of your food.

Eliminate drinking any sodas, coffee, tea or other drinks during your meals. If you need to clear your dry throat use a little water, which is a room temperature. Cold liquids will slow down your digestive processes.

Eating meals with more than one solid food such as meat and potatoes, chicken and rice, fish and rice, chicken and noodles, eggs and toast, cheese and bread will diminish the energy you need during the elimination cycle 1.

It is permissible to eat beef and chicken at the same time but not chicken and eggs or beef and nuts or chicken and beans. Eat the same type of protein at the same time but do not mix different proteins.

It's ok to eat different types of carbohydrates at the same time, with a salad, but not with protein, since carbohydrates digest easier than protein.

Eating a protein and a carbohydrate at the same time sets the stage for severe illness later in life. A protein requires acid for digestion and a carbohydrate requires alkaline juices for digestion.

This combination produces acid juices and alkaline juices at the same time. This combination produces water, which creates digestive juices that cannot fully digest either type of food.

In this case, the body produces more acid and more alkaline juices, which again are neutralized. The cycle continues until the food in your stomach starts to putrefy and ferment causing gas and acids. The gas causes belching and the combination gas and acids can lead to acid reflux.

As foods turn into acids because of the putrefaction and fermentation process, this acid food spoils all of the food in your stomach, causing undigested food to back flow up your esophagus and flow prematurely into your small intestine.

Food that is partially undigested becomes acidic, which affect the health of your colon, and when absorbed into your body is converted into fat and stored as a toxin your body.

In many cases the fermentation of food results in the production of alcohol and is similar to a person who drinks alcohol. There have been cases where people have been arrested for drunk driving and have never drank in their life and they wonder why they had a high blood alcohol level.

Eating the right combinations of foods at mealtime helps to preserve your energy for the elimination cycle and prevents you from creating spoiled food in your stomach that is converted to acid waste.

It is this acid waste that results in illness and fat. This is the reason most people as they age come down with various illnesses that terminate their life early or gain excessive weight.

Natural Body Cycle 3

Cycle 3 is the assimilation cycle and is from 8pm to 4am. This is the time the food you have eaten during the day is assimilated, absorbed and distributed throughout your body through your blood.

Food that was eaten during cycle II and that was combined and eaten properly will digest within 3 to 4 hours. Whereas food not combine properly, a meal consisting of protein and carbohydrates, can take up to 8 hours to pass through the stomach. During this time, your food will putrefy and ferment and become acidic. Under these conditions you will not get a lot of nutrients from that meal.

Eat your last meal by 6-7pm so that your food digests in your stomach by the time you go to bed. After three hours later, your food will have moved into your small intestine where it is ready for assimilation

When you go to bed 3 hours after your last meal, the next 6 hours, until 4am, your body will be absorbing the food you have eaten the previous day.

Remember, anything you do different than what these cycles call for will disrupt them and cause them to become extended. When this happens, your food turns into acid, you don't absorb   the value of your food, you lose energy and become tired, and over time you gain weight and create serious illnesses.

Have you ever notices how everyone you know eventually comes down with some sickness, which require surgery or doctor's drugs. Think about it. Is this what you want happening to you? Just start changing your eating habits slowly and as time passes you will be doing more and more of what your body's natural cycles need.

Chapter 10: How to do a Fast Body Cleanse

In any health program, the first thing you need to do is a colon cleanse. Once you do this, whatever health program you start, you will get the maximum benefits of that program. To keep good health, you need to make sure you have regular bowel movements. If you are not regular, you will have a toxic colon that will be supplying toxicity to all parts of your body.

If you eat 3 meals each day, you should have at least 2 bowel movements a day. If you only have one, then you are short 1 bowel movement.

Normally, if you have 3 full meals each day, you should have 3 bowel movements a day. Don't be fooled by anyone that says one bowel movement in one or two days is ok. This is not true.

If you want to learn how to keep regular using natural remedies, than you can check out my e-book called,

"Constipation Natural Cures" Look for it on Google Search or get The Best Constipation Remedies kindle e-book.

Here is a colon cleanse you can do with fruits and vegetable for a 3 day cleanse.

So let's get started.

To get your bowels moving like they should, you need to clean out what is in your colon right now. So the first day is for cleaning out your colon. The next two days are for cleaning the colon and detoxifying your body.

Doing a colon cleanse a minimum of three days is the best way to start cleaning out the colon, to detoxify the blood, and rejuvenate your body. Just doing a cleanse for three days is not a cure all and it will require more work after, on your part by starting to eat more natural foods.

The 3 day cleanse is a mini-fruit juice cleanse. You can do this juice fast once a month or every 6 months for 2-3 days, but leave out the prune juice and just drink the juices for 2-3 days. This gives your stomach, small and large intestine, and liver a rest and a chance to rejuvenate.

Doing a juice cleanse can give you some side effects where you feel nausea or slightly sick. Not everyone will get these effects.

This three day colon cleansing is outlined in my "Colon And Blood Cleansing Diet." In kindle form.

In her extensive book, Cooking For Healthy Healing, 1991, Linda Rector-page, N.D., Ph.D., talks about what a fast does,

"Fasting works by self-digestion. During a cleanse, the body in its infinite wisdom, will decompose and burn only the substances and tissue that are damaged, diseased, or unneeded, such as abscesses, tumors, excess fat deposits, and congestive wastes. Even a relatively short fast can accelerate elimination from the liver, kidneys, lungs and skin, often causing dramatic changes as masses of accumulated waste is expelled. Live foods and juices can literally pick up dead matter from the body and carry it away."

Day before the fast

The day before the fast, eat a large salad and two apples. This will give you plenty of fiber to scrub the walls of your colon as you move fecal matter out of your colon the following day.

First day of colon cleanse

Do this cleanse on a Saturday, Sunday or any other day that you don't have to go anywhere. You will be going to the bathroom all day and at times you need to be there quick.

Buy the following items.

- Organic apple juice – one gallon
- Organic apples – 6 for one day
- Organic prune juice – one quart

When you first wake up in the morning, you start by drinking 8 oz. of prune juice. Then, 10 minutes later, drink another 8oz of prune juice, and finally, 10 minutes later again drink another 8 oz. of prune juice.

Now, wait 20 minutes then drink 8 oz. of apple juice. Now, wait 30 minutes than drink another 8 oz. of apple juice

If you haven't sped to the bathroom yet, you will in a little while.

Now you will be drinking 8 oz. of apple juice every hour until the end of the day. You can stop drinking apple juice around 5pm.

During the day, you can eat three apples in the morning and 3 apples in the evening.

This process will clean out any fecal matter that has been sitting your colon for days and gets you ready for the next step.

Second way to start the colon cleanse

Another way to start a colon cleanse is to use a product that is called "Oxy-Powder." This product is in capsules and is used for 30 days. Simply by taking capsules every day, you will clean out your colon and any build up along your colon walls.

This is a very effective product and will send you to the bathroom frequently as it clean out your colon. Start this cleanse on a Saturday so you can have Saturday and Sunday free to start cleaning out your colon. For a gentle cleanse you can start with about 4 Oxy-Powder capsules. Ten capsules will surely send you to the bathroom frequently. Take the capsules the night before you start your cleanse.

After two days of intense cleaning, you can back off and continue to take a lower number of capsules to continue your cleanse at a slower pace – 2 to 4 capsule per day. Oxy-powder is not a laxative and is not addictive. But, it will make your stools watery.

You can get Oxy-Powder on the internet.

Second day of the colon cleanse

During the second day you can drink different kinds of juices and eat 2-6 apples. You can drink any kind of juice be it fruit or vegetable. A combination of fruit and vegetable juice is good.

Third day of the colon cleanse

The third day is like the second day where you can drink different kinds of juices and eat 2-6 apples or other fruits. You can drink any kind of juice be it fruit or vegetable. A combination of fruit and vegetable juice is good

Fourth Day, after the fast is done

After you have finished your three-day fast, start eating soft foods to gently adjust your system to food. Here are some of the foods you can eat during the fourth day out of your fast,

Baked potato

Fruit salad

Fruit smoothie

Light soup

Oatmeal, multigrain cereal with banana

Salad

Natural Yogurt

CHAPTER 11: RESOURCES YOU NEED TO KNOW ABOUT

Rudy Silva is a natural consultant nutritionist educated in the United State in Nutrition and Physics. He is a graduate from the San Jose State University in California. He is author of 30 other e-books on natural remedies. He has authored a newsletter in natural remedies for over 4 years. He has many websites promoting special recommended products and information.

Resource page

Here are some of the other kindle e-books about natural remedies that have been written by this author. You can see the entire list at:

http://tinyurl.com/b2f7wd3

Acne Remedies
Best natural acne treatments: Acne facial

Constipation Remedies
Best Constipated Women Natural Cures
How To Relieve Constipation With Fruits

Essential Fatty Acids
Taking The Mystery Out Of Essential Fatty acids

Men's Health
Best Impotence Health Diet

Weight loss
Ten (10) Day Quick Success Weight Loss Program: A new approach to losing weight by changing your eating habits for life

To see all of the kindle books written by this author, go to this the Authors Profile Page or this URL:

http://tinyurl.com/b2f7wd3

If you need support or want to promote any of his e-books, please contact him at rss41@yahoo.com and expect a reply within 24 hours. He looks forward to hearing from you and is happy to help you understand his material on natural and nutritional health.

Give A Review

And, don't for get to give a review for this e-book at Amazon so that others can gain the benefits of what is in this e-book.

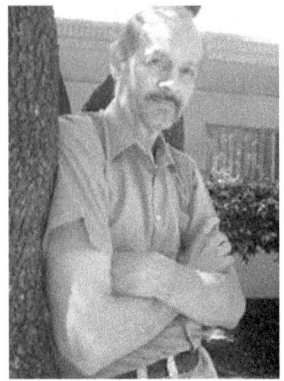

To you, for creating better health and more happiness in your life,

Rudy S Silva

www.ingramcontent.com/pod-product-compliance
Lightning Source LLC
Chambersburg PA
CBHW070708290526
45790CB00001B/495